CONTENTS

Chapter 1: Introduction to Esophagitis — 1

Chapter 2: Anatomy and Physiology of the Esophagus — 23

Chapter 3: Gastroesophageal Reflux Disease (GERD) and Esophagitis — 40

Chapter 4: Infectious Esophagitis — 59

Chapter 5: Eosinophilic Esophagitis (EoE) — 73

Chapter 6: Chemical and Drug-Induced Esophagitis — 92

Chapter 7: Radiation Esophagitis — 115

Chapter 8: Refractory Esophagitis and Complications — 132

Chapter 9: Diagnostic Approaches in Esophagitis — 148

Chapter 10: Pharmacological Management of Esophagitis — 160

Chapter 11: Non-Pharmacological Interventions and Lifestyle Modifications — 172

Chapter 12: Integrative and Holistic Approaches to Esophagitis Management — 185

Chapter 13: Surgical Management of Esophagitis and Refractory Cases — 192

CHAPTER 1: INTRODUCTION TO ESOPHAGITIS

Definition and Overview

Esophagitis, derived from the Greek words "oesophagus" (meaning "gullet" or "tube") and "-itis" (denoting inflammation), refers to the inflammation of the esophageal mucosa, the inner lining of the esophagus. This condition can result from a variety of causes, leading to discomfort, pain, and potential complications. Understanding the definition and overview of esophagitis is crucial for elucidating its complexities and developing effective management strategies.

The esophagus is a muscular tube approximately 25 centimeters in length, extending from the pharynx to the stomach. Its primary function is to transport swallowed food and liquids from the mouth to the stomach through a series of coordinated muscle contractions known as peristalsis. The esophageal mucosa consists of several layers, including the epithelium, lamina propria, and muscularis mucosae, which collectively provide protection and facilitate the movement of ingested material.

Esophagitis occurs when the delicate balance of the esophageal mucosal barrier is disrupted, leading to inflammation and injury. This disruption can result from various factors, including gastroesophageal reflux disease (GERD), infections, chemical irritants, radiation therapy, and autoimmune conditions. Each etiology of esophagitis presents unique challenges in diagnosis and management, highlighting the importance of a comprehensive approach to patient care.

The clinical presentation of esophagitis can vary widely depending on the underlying cause and severity of inflammation. Common symptoms include dysphagia (difficulty swallowing), odynophagia (painful swallowing), retrosternal chest pain, heartburn, regurgitation, and nausea. Patients may also experience complications such as esophageal strictures, ulceration, bleeding, and perforation, which can have serious implications for their health and quality of life.

Diagnosing esophagitis typically involves a combination of clinical evaluation, endoscopic examination, histopathological analysis, and ancillary testing. Endoscopy allows for direct visualization of the esophageal mucosa, enabling the detection of inflammation, erosions, ulcers, strictures, and other abnormalities. Biopsy specimens obtained during endoscopy can provide valuable information regarding the underlying histopathology and etiology of esophagitis, guiding appropriate treatment decisions.

Treatment strategies for esophagitis aim to alleviate symptoms, promote healing, and prevent complications. Pharmacological interventions often play a central role and may include acid-suppressive medications such as proton pump inhibitors (PPIs), histamine-2 receptor antagonists (H2RAs), mucosal protectants, anti-inflammatory agents, and immunomodulatory drugs. In addition to pharmacotherapy, non-pharmacological interventions such as lifestyle modifications, dietary changes, and behavioral therapies are also important components of comprehensive management plans.

Holistic approaches to esophagitis management recognize the interconnectedness of physical, psychological, and social factors that influence health and well-being. Integrative therapies such as herbal medicine, acupuncture, yoga, and mindfulness-based stress reduction techniques can complement conventional treatments, providing patients with a holistic framework for healing and self-care. By addressing the underlying causes of inflammation and supporting the body's innate healing mechanisms, holistic approaches seek to optimize patient outcomes and enhance overall quality of life.

In summary, esophagitis is a multifaceted condition characterized by inflammation of the esophageal mucosa, which can result from various etiologies and present with diverse clinical manifestations. A thorough understanding of the definition and overview of esophagitis is essential for clinicians to recognize, diagnose, and manage this condition effectively. By employing a multidisciplinary approach that integrates pharmacological, non-pharmacological, and holistic interventions, clinicians can provide comprehensive care that addresses the complex needs of patients with esophagitis.

Epidemiology and Prevalence

Understanding the epidemiology and prevalence of esophagitis is essential for assessing its public health impact, identifying at-risk populations, and guiding preventive and therapeutic interventions. Epidemiological studies provide valuable insights into the incidence, prevalence, risk factors, and geographic variations of esophagitis, shedding light on its burden and distribution across different populations and regions.

Esophagitis is a common gastrointestinal disorder with a significant global prevalence, affecting individuals of all ages and demographics. While precise epidemiological data can vary depending on the definition, diagnostic criteria, and study population, several key trends and patterns have emerged from population-based surveys, cohort studies, and systematic reviews.

Gastroesophageal reflux disease (GERD) is the leading cause of esophagitis, accounting for a substantial proportion of cases worldwide. GERD is characterized by the reflux of gastric contents into the esophagus due to dysfunction of the lower esophageal sphincter (LES) or impaired esophageal clearance mechanisms. Chronic exposure to gastric acid, bile acids, and pepsin can lead to mucosal inflammation, erosion, and ulceration, predisposing individuals to the development of esophagitis.

The prevalence of GERD and GERD-related esophagitis has been increasing in many parts of the world, particularly in Western countries where lifestyle factors such as obesity, dietary habits, and tobacco use are prevalent. Population-based studies have reported a wide range of prevalence estimates for GERD, ranging from 10% to 40% in North America and Europe, with lower rates observed in Asian and African populations.

In addition to GERD, infectious esophagitis represents another significant etiology of esophageal inflammation, particularly in immunocompromised individuals such as those with HIV/AIDS, organ transplant recipients, and patients undergoing chemotherapy or immunosuppressive therapy. Opportunistic pathogens such as Candida albicans, herpes simplex virus (HSV), cytomegalovirus (CMV), and human papillomavirus (HPV) can cause esophagitis in susceptible hosts, leading to significant morbidity and mortality if left untreated.

The prevalence of infectious esophagitis varies depending on the underlying immunodeficiency, exposure to pathogens, and healthcare settings. For example, Candida esophagitis is one of the most common opportunistic infections in patients with HIV/AIDS, affecting up to 20% to 40% of individuals with advanced immunosuppression. Conversely, CMV esophagitis is more commonly observed in transplant recipients and patients receiving high-dose corticosteroids or immunosuppressive medications.

Eosinophilic esophagitis (EoE) is a chronic immune-mediated disorder characterized by eosinophilic infiltration of the esophageal mucosa, resulting in dysphagia, food impaction, and esophageal strictures. EoE has emerged as a significant cause of esophagitis, particularly in pediatric and young adult populations, although its prevalence appears to be increasing across all age groups. Population-based studies have reported EoE prevalence estimates ranging from 0.5 to 1 per 1,000 individuals in Western countries, with higher rates observed in regions with greater awareness and diagnostic expertise.

Chemical and drug-induced esophagitis can occur secondary to the ingestion of corrosive substances, medications, or toxic agents that damage the esophageal mucosa. Common culprits include nonsteroidal anti-inflammatory drugs (NSAIDs), bisphosphonates, potassium supplements, and certain antibiotics. The prevalence of drug-induced esophagitis varies depending on the frequency of medication use, formulation, and patient factors such as age, comorbidities, and concomitant medications.

Radiation esophagitis is another important consideration, particularly in patients undergoing thoracic radiation therapy for malignancies such as lung cancer, esophageal cancer, and lymphomas. Radiation-induced injury to the esophageal mucosa can lead to acute and chronic inflammation, ulceration, strictures, and perforation, resulting in significant morbidity and impairing quality of life. The prevalence of radiation esophagitis depends on factors such as radiation dose, fractionation, target volume, and concurrent chemotherapy, with rates ranging from 15% to 40% in clinical studies.

Refractory esophagitis, defined as persistent or recurrent inflammation despite optimal medical or surgical therapy, represents a challenging subset of cases that require specialized management. Refractory esophagitis can result from various factors, including inadequate acid suppression, treatment nonadherence, persistent underlying pathology, and complications such as strictures or Barrett's esophagus. The prevalence of refractory esophagitis is not well-defined and may vary depending on the population studied and the criteria used to define refractoriness.

In summary, esophagitis encompasses a diverse range of inflammatory conditions affecting the esophageal mucosa, with varying etiologies, clinical presentations, and epidemiological patterns. While GERD remains the most common cause of esophagitis globally, infectious, eosinophilic, chemical, drug-induced, and radiation-induced esophagitis are also significant contributors to the overall burden of disease. Understanding the epidemiology and prevalence of esophagitis is essential for informing public health initiatives, guiding clinical practice, and improving patient outcomes. Further research is needed to elucidate the evolving epidemiology of esophagitis and identify opportunities for prevention, early detection, and targeted intervention.

Etiology and Risk Factors

Etiology and risk factors play a critical role in the development and progression of esophagitis, influencing its pathogenesis, clinical presentation, and treatment outcomes. Understanding the underlying causes and predisposing factors associated with esophageal inflammation is essential for targeted prevention, early detection, and effective management strategies.

Gastroesophageal Reflux Disease (GERD):

GERD is the leading cause of esophagitis, accounting for a significant proportion of cases worldwide. It is characterized by the reflux of gastric contents, including acid, bile acids, and pepsin, into the esophagus due to dysfunction of the lower esophageal sphincter (LES) or impaired esophageal clearance mechanisms. Chronic exposure to gastric refluxate can lead to mucosal injury, inflammation, erosion, and ulceration, resulting in GERD-associated esophagitis.

Risk Factors for GERD-associated Esophagitis:

- Obesity: Increased intra-abdominal pressure and adipose tissue contribute to LES dysfunction and promote reflux.
- Hiatal Hernia: Displacement of the stomach into the thoracic cavity disrupts the gastroesophageal junction and impairs esophageal clearance.
- Dietary Factors: High-fat foods, spicy foods, citrus fruits, caffeine, and alcohol can exacerbate reflux symptoms.
- Tobacco Use: Smoking weakens the LES and impairs esophageal motility, predisposing individuals to reflux.
- Pregnancy: Hormonal changes and increased intra-abdominal pressure during pregnancy can exacerbate GERD symptoms.

Infectious Esophagitis:

Infectious esophagitis results from the invasion of the esophageal mucosa by pathogens such as Candida albicans, herpes simplex virus (HSV), cytomegalovirus (CMV), and human papillomavirus (HPV). Immunocompromised individuals, including those with HIV/AIDS, organ transplant recipients, and patients undergoing chemotherapy or immunosuppressive therapy, are particularly susceptible to opportunistic infections.

Risk Factors for Infectious Esophagitis:

- Immunodeficiency: Impaired cell-mediated immunity predisposes individuals to opportunistic infections, especially Candida esophagitis in patients with HIV/AIDS.
- Chemotherapy: Cytotoxic drugs can suppress the immune system and increase susceptibility to viral and fungal infections.
- Immunosuppressive Therapy: Agents such as corticosteroids, calcineurin inhibitors, and antimetabolites can weaken immune defenses and promote pathogen proliferation.
- HIV/AIDS: Human immunodeficiency virus (HIV) infection leads to CD4+ T-cell depletion and increases the risk of opportunistic infections, including esophagitis.

Eosinophilic Esophagitis (EoE):

EoE is a chronic immune-mediated disorder characterized by eosinophilic infiltration of the esophageal mucosa, resulting in dysphagia, food impaction, and esophageal strictures. Although the exact etiology of EoE remains unclear, it is thought to involve a complex interplay between genetic predisposition, environmental triggers, and immune dysregulation.

Risk Factors for EoE:

- Atopic Conditions: EoE is commonly associated with allergic diseases such as asthma, allergic rhinitis, and atopic dermatitis, suggesting a shared pathophysiological mechanism.
- Food Allergens: Sensitization to dietary antigens, particularly milk, eggs, soy, wheat, and nuts, may trigger eosinophilic inflammation in the esophagus.
- Aeroallergens: Exposure to airborne allergens such as pollen, dust mites, and animal dander may exacerbate EoE symptoms in susceptible individuals.
- Genetic Predisposition: Family history of EoE and genetic variants in genes related to epithelial barrier function, immune regulation, and allergic inflammation may increase susceptibility to the disease.

Chemical and Drug-Induced Esophagitis:

Chemical and drug-induced esophagitis can occur secondary to the ingestion of corrosive substances, medications, or toxic agents that damage the esophageal mucosa. Common culprits include nonsteroidal anti-inflammatory drugs (NSAIDs), bisphosphonates, potassium supplements, and certain antibiotics.

Risk Factors for Chemical and Drug-Induced Esophagitis:

- Medication Use: Prolonged or frequent use of medications with esophageal irritant properties, such as NSAIDs and bisphosphonates, increases the risk of drug-induced esophagitis.
- Potassium Supplements: Oral potassium supplements, particularly in solid tablet form, can cause esophageal ulceration and stricture formation if not taken with

adequate water or while lying down.
- Pill Esophagitis: Difficulty swallowing or improper administration of medications, especially large or poorly lubricated pills, can lead to mucosal injury and esophageal inflammation.

Radiation Esophagitis:

Radiation esophagitis occurs as a consequence of thoracic radiation therapy for malignancies such as lung cancer, esophageal cancer, and lymphomas. Radiation-induced injury to the esophageal mucosa can manifest as acute or chronic inflammation, ulceration, strictures, and perforation, resulting in significant morbidity and impaired quality of life.

Risk Factors for Radiation Esophagitis:

- Radiation Dose and Volume: Higher radiation doses and larger target volumes increase the risk of radiation-induced esophageal toxicity.
- Concurrent Chemotherapy: Combined modality therapy with chemotherapy and radiation may potentiate esophageal injury and exacerbate acute and late toxicities.
- Patient Factors: Age, comorbidities, performance status, smoking history, and preexisting esophageal pathology influence individual susceptibility to radiation-induced esophagitis.

Refractory Esophagitis:

Refractory esophagitis refers to persistent or recurrent inflammation despite optimal medical or surgical therapy, posing diagnostic and therapeutic challenges for clinicians. Various factors may contribute to treatment resistance, including inadequate acid suppression, treatment nonadherence, persistent underlying pathology, and complications such as strictures or Barrett's esophagus.

Risk Factors for Refractory Esophagitis:

- Inadequate Acid Suppression: Suboptimal dosing, poor compliance, nocturnal acid breakthrough, and proton pump inhibitor (PPI) resistance can compromise acid suppression and exacerbate esophageal inflammation.
- Treatment Nonadherence: Failure to adhere to prescribed medications, dietary restrictions, and lifestyle modifications can undermine therapeutic efficacy and contribute to treatment failure.
- Persistent Pathology: Persistent underlying pathology, such as severe erosive esophagitis, Barrett's esophagus, or eosinophilic inflammation, may require aggressive treatment strategies to achieve remission.
- Complications: Complications such as esophageal strictures, ulcerations, and Barrett's esophagus may necessitate additional interventions, including endoscopic dilation, mucosal resection, or surgical intervention.

In summary, esophagitis encompasses a diverse spectrum of inflammatory conditions affecting the esophageal mucosa, with multifactorial etiologies and complex interactions between genetic, environmental, and host factors. Gastroesophageal reflux disease (GERD), infectious agents, eosinophilic inflammation, chemical and drug exposures, radiation therapy, and refractory disease represent important contributors to the pathogenesis of esophagitis, highlighting the need for comprehensive risk assessment, targeted prevention, and individualized management strategies. By addressing underlying etiologies and modifying predisposing factors, clinicians can optimize outcomes and improve the quality of life for patients with esophagitis.

Pathophysiology

The pathophysiology of esophagitis encompasses a complex interplay of molecular, cellular, and physiological processes that contribute to inflammation, injury, and tissue remodeling within the esophageal mucosa. Understanding the underlying mechanisms driving esophageal inflammation is crucial for elucidating disease pathogenesis, identifying therapeutic targets, and guiding the development of effective management strategies.

Gastroesophageal Reflux Disease (GERD)-Associated Esophagitis:

In the context of GERD, esophagitis develops as a consequence of repeated exposure of the esophageal mucosa to gastric contents, including acid, bile acids, and pepsin. Dysfunction of the lower esophageal sphincter (LES) and impaired esophageal clearance mechanisms allow for retrograde flow of gastric refluxate into the esophagus, leading to mucosal injury and inflammation.

Key Pathophysiological Mechanisms of GERD-Associated Esophagitis:

1. **LES Dysfunction:** Reduced resting tone and transient relaxation of the LES permit reflux of gastric contents into the esophagus, promoting mucosal exposure to acidic and injurious substances.
2. **Impaired Esophageal Clearance:** Defects in peristalsis, ineffective esophageal motility, and delayed gastric emptying contribute to prolonged contact time

between refluxate and the esophageal mucosa.
3. **Acidic Injury:** Hydrochloric acid (HCl) is a major component of gastric refluxate and is highly corrosive to the esophageal epithelium, causing direct mucosal damage and inflammation.
4. **Bile Acid Exposure:** Bile acids, particularly in the presence of alkaline pH, can further exacerbate mucosal injury by disrupting epithelial barrier function, inducing oxidative stress, and activating inflammatory pathways.
5. **Pepsin Activation:** Pepsin, a proteolytic enzyme secreted by gastric chief cells, is activated by acidic pH and can digest esophageal proteins, leading to tissue injury and triggering immune responses.

Infectious Esophagitis:

Infectious esophagitis results from the invasion of the esophageal mucosa by pathogens such as Candida albicans, herpes simplex virus (HSV), cytomegalovirus (CMV), and human papillomavirus (HPV). These microorganisms can cause direct tissue damage, induce inflammation, and elicit host immune responses that contribute to esophageal injury and dysfunction.

Pathophysiological Mechanisms of Infectious Esophagitis:

1. **Microbial Invasion:** Pathogens such as Candida, HSV, CMV, and HPV can directly invade esophageal epithelial cells, leading to cell lysis, ulceration, and tissue destruction.
2. **Inflammatory Response:** Host immune cells, including neutrophils, macrophages, and lymphocytes, are recruited to the site of infection, resulting in local inflammation, edema, and tissue injury.
3. **Immune Dysregulation:** In immunocompromised

individuals, impaired cell-mediated immunity and deficient mucosal defenses predispose to opportunistic infections and facilitate pathogen colonization and dissemination.
4. **Viral Latency and Reactivation:** Herpesviruses such as HSV and CMV can establish latent infections within sensory ganglia or lymphoid tissues and undergo periodic reactivation, leading to recurrent episodes of esophagitis in susceptible hosts.

Eosinophilic Esophagitis (EoE):

EoE is characterized by eosinophilic infiltration of the esophageal mucosa, resulting in dysphagia, food impaction, and esophageal strictures. The pathogenesis of EoE involves a complex interplay between genetic predisposition, environmental triggers, allergen exposure, and immune dysregulation.

Key Pathophysiological Mechanisms of EoE:

1. **Allergic Sensitization:** Sensitization to dietary antigens and environmental allergens triggers activation of the adaptive immune system, leading to Th2-mediated immune responses and eosinophil recruitment to the esophageal mucosa.
2. **Eosinophilic Inflammation:** Eosinophils release proinflammatory cytokines, chemokines, and cytotoxic granule proteins that promote tissue inflammation, epithelial injury, and remodeling.
3. **Epithelial Barrier Dysfunction:** Impaired epithelial barrier function, characterized by alterations in tight junction proteins and mucin expression, facilitates allergen penetration and antigen presentation, perpetuating immune activation and inflammation.
4. **Dysregulated Immune Responses:** Dysregulation of

immune checkpoints, including PD-1/PD-L1 and CTLA-4 pathways, may contribute to aberrant immune activation and perpetuate eosinophilic inflammation in EoE.

Chemical and Drug-Induced Esophagitis:

Chemical and drug-induced esophagitis can occur secondary to the ingestion of corrosive substances, medications, or toxic agents that damage the esophageal mucosa. These insults disrupt mucosal integrity, induce cellular injury, and elicit inflammatory responses within the esophageal epithelium.

Pathophysiological Mechanisms of Chemical and Drug-Induced Esophagitis:

1. **Direct Mucosal Injury:** Corrosive substances such as strong acids, alkalis, and caustic agents cause direct chemical injury to the esophageal epithelium, leading to mucosal necrosis, ulceration, and hemorrhage.
2. **Local Irritation:** Irritant medications such as nonsteroidal anti-inflammatory drugs (NSAIDs), bisphosphonates, and potassium supplements can irritate the esophageal mucosa, induce local inflammation, and impair mucosal healing.
3. **Local pH Changes:** Acidic or alkaline medications can alter the pH of esophageal luminal contents, disrupting mucosal pH homeostasis, and promoting epithelial injury and inflammation.
4. **Tablet-Induced Injury:** Large or poorly lubricated pills can lodge in the esophageal lumen, cause mechanical abrasion or frictional injury to the mucosa, and trigger inflammatory responses.

Radiation Esophagitis:

Radiation esophagitis occurs as a consequence of thoracic

radiation therapy for malignancies such as lung cancer, esophageal cancer, and lymphomas. Radiation-induced injury to the esophageal mucosa leads to acute and chronic inflammation, epithelial damage, and fibrotic remodeling of the esophageal wall.

Pathophysiological Mechanisms of Radiation Esophagitis:

1. **DNA Damage:** Ionizing radiation generates free radicals and induces DNA strand breaks, leading to cellular injury, apoptosis, and necrosis within the esophageal epithelium.
2. **Inflammatory Responses:** Radiation triggers release of proinflammatory cytokines, chemokines, and growth factors that recruit immune cells, promote tissue inflammation, and amplify tissue injury.
3. **Vascular Injury:** Radiation disrupts the microvascular architecture of the esophageal wall, causing endothelial damage, capillary leakage, and tissue hypoxia, which further exacerbate inflammation and impair wound healing.
4. **Fibrotic Remodeling:** Chronic radiation exposure stimulates fibroblast activation, collagen deposition, and extracellular matrix remodeling, leading to esophageal fibrosis, stricture formation, and functional impairment.

Refractory Esophagitis:

Refractory esophagitis refers to persistent or recurrent inflammation despite optimal medical or surgical therapy, posing diagnostic and therapeutic challenges for clinicians. The pathophysiology of refractory esophagitis may involve underlying disease mechanisms such as persistent acid reflux, ongoing mucosal injury, impaired tissue healing, or treatment resistance.

Key Pathophysiological Mechanisms of Refractory Esophagitis:

1. **Inadequate Acid Suppression:** Suboptimal acid suppression, nocturnal acid breakthrough, and PPI resistance can perpetuate mucosal inflammation and compromise treatment efficacy in GERD-associated esophagitis.
2. **Persistent Underlying Pathology:** Incomplete resolution of underlying disease processes, such as eosinophilic inflammation in EoE or infectious agents in infectious esophagitis, may contribute to treatment failure and disease recurrence.
3. **Complications:** Structural complications such as esophageal strictures, ulcerations, and Barrett's esophagus may necessitate additional interventions, including endoscopic dilation, mucosal resection, or surgical intervention, to achieve symptom relief and mucosal healing.

In summary, the pathophysiology of esophagitis is characterized by a complex interplay of molecular, cellular, and physiological processes that contribute to mucosal inflammation, injury, and tissue remodeling within the esophageal mucosa. Gastroesophageal reflux disease (GERD), infectious agents, eosinophilic inflammation, chemical and drug exposures, radiation therapy, and refractory disease represent important etiological factors that drive esophageal inflammation and dysfunction. By elucidating the underlying mechanisms driving esophageal inflammation, clinicians can develop targeted therapeutic strategies aimed at mitigating mucosal injury, promoting tissue healing, and improving patient outcomes.

Classification and Types

Esophagitis encompasses a diverse spectrum of inflammatory conditions affecting the esophageal mucosa, each with distinct etiologies, clinical presentations, histopathological features, and management approaches. Classification systems based on underlying mechanisms, histological findings, endoscopic features, and clinical criteria provide valuable frameworks for characterizing esophageal inflammation and guiding diagnostic and therapeutic decisions.

Classification Based on Etiology:

1. **Gastroesophageal Reflux Disease (GERD)-Associated Esophagitis:**

GERD-associated esophagitis results from chronic exposure of the esophageal mucosa to gastric refluxate, including acid, bile acids, and pepsin, due to dysfunction of the lower esophageal sphincter (LES) or impaired esophageal clearance mechanisms.

Subtypes of GERD-associated esophagitis may include erosive esophagitis, characterized by visible mucosal erosions or ulcers on endoscopy, and nonerosive reflux disease (NERD), characterized by symptomatic reflux in the absence of visible mucosal injury.

2. **Infectious Esophagitis:**

Infectious esophagitis results from the invasion of the esophageal mucosa by pathogens such as Candida albicans, herpes simplex virus (HSV), cytomegalovirus (CMV), and human papillomavirus (HPV).

Subtypes of infectious esophagitis may include Candida esophagitis, HSV esophagitis, CMV esophagitis, and HPV-related esophageal lesions, each with characteristic clinical presentations, endoscopic findings, and histopathological features.

3. Eosinophilic Esophagitis (EoE):

EoE is a chronic immune-mediated disorder characterized by eosinophilic infiltration of the esophageal mucosa, leading to dysphagia, food impaction, and esophageal strictures.

Subtypes of EoE may include active eosinophilic inflammation, fibrostenotic disease with esophageal strictures, and inactive disease with histological remission but persistent symptoms.

4. Chemical and Drug-Induced Esophagitis:

Chemical and drug-induced esophagitis can occur secondary to the ingestion of corrosive substances, medications, or toxic agents that damage the esophageal mucosa.

Subtypes of drug-induced esophagitis may include NSAID-induced esophagitis, bisphosphonate-associated esophagitis, and potassium-induced ulcerative esophagitis, each with specific risk factors and clinical features.

5. Radiation Esophagitis:

Radiation esophagitis occurs as a consequence of thoracic radiation therapy for malignancies such as lung cancer, esophageal cancer, and lymphomas.

Subtypes of radiation esophagitis may include acute radiation esophagitis, characterized by transient mucosal inflammation and dysphagia, and chronic radiation esophagitis, characterized by fibrotic remodeling and long-term complications such as strictures and dysphagia.

Classification Based on Endoscopic Findings:

1. Erosive Esophagitis:

Erosive esophagitis is characterized by visible mucosal erosions or ulcers on endoscopy, typically located in the distal esophagus. The severity of erosive esophagitis may be graded using the Los Angeles Classification system, which categorizes lesions based on the extent of mucosal involvement and the presence of complications such as strictures.

2. **Nonerosive Reflux Disease (NERD):**

NERD refers to symptomatic reflux in the absence of visible mucosal injury on endoscopy.

Diagnosis of NERD may require additional testing, such as esophageal pH monitoring or impedance-pH testing, to confirm abnormal esophageal acid exposure or reflux events.

3. **Candida Esophagitis:**

Candida esophagitis is characterized by white or yellowish plaques, pseudomembranes, or friable mucosa on endoscopic examination, often associated with underlying immunodeficiency or immunosuppressive therapy.

4. **Herpes Simplex Virus (HSV) Esophagitis:**

HSV esophagitis typically presents with linear or serpiginous ulcers, discrete vesicles, or hemorrhagic plaques on endoscopy, particularly in immunocompromised individuals.

5. **Cytomegalovirus (CMV) Esophagitis:**

CMV esophagitis may manifest as shallow or deep ulcers, linear fissures, or pseudomembranes on endoscopy, often accompanied by systemic symptoms and evidence of CMV viremia.

6. **Eosinophilic Esophagitis (EoE):**

EoE is characterized by features such as linear furrows, concentric rings, white exudates, mucosal edema, and strictures on endoscopic examination, often with normal or subtle mucosal changes visible to the naked eye.

7. **Drug-Induced Esophagitis:**

Drug-induced esophagitis may present with features such as localized or diffuse erosions, ulcers, or strictures on endoscopy, typically corresponding to the site of drug contact within the esophagus.

Classification Based on Histopathological Findings:

1. **Erosive Esophagitis:**

Histological features of erosive esophagitis may include neutrophilic infiltration, basal cell hyperplasia, loss of surface epithelium, and evidence of acute or chronic inflammation on biopsy.

2. **Eosinophilic Esophagitis (EoE):**

Histopathological findings in EoE typically include eosinophilic infiltration of the esophageal mucosa, eosinophilic microabscesses, basal zone hyperplasia, papillary elongation, and dilated intercellular spaces.

3. **Infectious Esophagitis:**

Histopathological features of infectious esophagitis may include viral cytopathic changes, intranuclear or intracytoplasmic inclusions, fungal hyphae, pseudohyphae, or viral inclusion bodies on biopsy.

Clinical Classification Based on Symptom Severity:

1. **Mild Esophagitis:**

Mild esophagitis may present with mild or intermittent symptoms such as heartburn, regurgitation, dysphagia, or chest pain, without evidence of mucosal injury or structural complications on endoscopy.

2. **Moderate Esophagitis:**

Moderate esophagitis may manifest with more frequent or persistent symptoms, moderate mucosal inflammation or erosions on endoscopy, and variable histological changes on biopsy.

3. **Severe Esophagitis:**

Severe esophagitis is characterized by severe or refractory symptoms, extensive mucosal erosions or ulcers, and significant histopathological changes such as marked eosinophilic infiltration or deep ulceration on biopsy.

In summary, esophagitis encompasses a diverse array of inflammatory conditions affecting the esophageal mucosa, each with unique etiologies, clinical manifestations, endoscopic features, histopathological findings, and management considerations. Classification systems based on underlying mechanisms, endoscopic findings, histological characteristics, and symptom severity provide valuable frameworks for characterizing esophageal inflammation and guiding diagnostic and therapeutic decisions tailored to individual patient needs. By understanding the classification and types of esophagitis, clinicians can effectively assess, diagnose, and manage patients with this heterogeneous group of disorders, optimizing patient care and outcomes.

CHAPTER 2: ANATOMY AND PHYSIOLOGY OF THE ESOPHAGUS

Structure and Function of the Esophagus

The esophagus is a tubular organ that forms part of the upper gastrointestinal tract, serving as a conduit for the transport of swallowed food and liquids from the pharynx to the stomach. Understanding the anatomical structure and physiological function of the esophagus is essential for comprehending its role in digestion, swallowing, and the pathogenesis of esophageal disorders.

Anatomical Structure:

The esophagus is approximately 25-30 centimeters (10-12 inches) in length and extends from the pharynx to the stomach. It consists of four main anatomical regions:

1. **Cervical Esophagus:** The uppermost portion of the

esophagus, located within the neck, extends from the inferior border of the cricoid cartilage to the superior border of the thoracic inlet. It is surrounded by the cervical vertebrae, trachea, and major vessels of the neck.
2. **Thoracic Esophagus:** The middle portion of the esophagus passes through the thoracic cavity, posterior to the trachea and heart, and anterior to the vertebral column. It descends along the posterior mediastinum, traversing the diaphragmatic hiatus to enter the abdominal cavity.
3. **Abdominal Esophagus:** The lowermost portion of the esophagus extends through the diaphragmatic hiatus into the abdominal cavity, where it connects to the cardiac orifice of the stomach. It is surrounded by the esophageal hiatus of the diaphragm and adjacent structures of the gastroesophageal junction.
4. **Gastroesophageal Junction (GEJ):** The transition zone between the distal esophagus and the proximal stomach, where the lower esophageal sphincter (LES) regulates the passage of food and prevents reflux of gastric contents into the esophagus.

Histological Layers:

The esophageal wall consists of several histological layers that provide structural support, facilitate motility, and protect against mechanical and chemical injury:

1. **Mucosa:** The innermost layer of the esophageal wall, composed of epithelial cells, lamina propria, and muscularis mucosae. The epithelium transitions from nonkeratinized stratified squamous epithelium in the upper esophagus to simple columnar epithelium in the lower esophagus near the GEJ.
2. **Submucosa:** The connective tissue layer beneath the

mucosa, containing blood vessels, lymphatics, nerves, and submucosal glands that secrete mucus to lubricate the esophageal lumen.
3. **Muscularis Propria:** The thick muscular layer responsible for peristaltic contractions that propel swallowed food and liquids through the esophagus. It consists of inner circular and outer longitudinal muscle layers that coordinate rhythmic contractions during swallowing.
4. **Adventitia or Serosa:** The outermost layer of the esophageal wall, composed of connective tissue and mesothelium, which anchors the esophagus to surrounding structures within the mediastinum or abdominal cavity.

Physiological Function:

The esophagus performs several key functions essential for the process of swallowing, digestion, and transit of food from the oral cavity to the stomach:

1. **Deglutition (Swallowing):** Swallowing is a complex neuromuscular process involving the coordinated contraction and relaxation of muscles in the oral cavity, pharynx, and esophagus. It consists of three sequential phases: oral (voluntary), pharyngeal (involuntary), and esophageal (involuntary).
2. **Peristalsis:** Peristalsis is the coordinated, sequential contraction of esophageal smooth muscle that propels swallowed food and liquids from the pharynx to the stomach. It is mediated by the enteric nervous system and controlled by neural reflexes involving the vagus nerve (cranial nerve X).
3. **Lower Esophageal Sphincter (LES) Function:** The LES is a specialized region of smooth muscle at the junction between the esophagus and stomach, which

maintains tonic contraction to prevent reflux of gastric contents into the esophagus during periods of rest and relaxation.

4. **Mucosal Protection:** The esophageal mucosa is equipped with several mechanisms to protect against mechanical and chemical injury from swallowed food, liquids, and gastric refluxate. These include the secretion of mucus by submucosal glands, rapid epithelial repair mechanisms, and sensory innervation to trigger protective reflexes.

Neurovascular Supply:

The esophagus receives its neurovascular supply from branches of the vagus nerve (cranial nerve X), sympathetic nerves from the thoracic splanchnic nerves, and blood vessels originating from the thoracic aorta and its branches. Parasympathetic innervation via the vagus nerve mediates esophageal peristalsis and LES relaxation, whereas sympathetic innervation modulates vascular tone and glandular secretion.

In summary, the esophagus is a tubular organ that forms part of the upper gastrointestinal tract, facilitating the transport of swallowed food and liquids from the pharynx to the stomach. Its anatomical structure, histological layers, physiological functions, and neurovascular supply collectively contribute to its role in digestion, swallowing, and protection against injury. Understanding the structure and function of the esophagus is essential for comprehending its normal physiology and the pathogenesis of esophageal disorders.

Mucosal Barrier and Defense Mechanisms

The esophageal mucosal barrier plays a crucial role in protecting the underlying tissues from mechanical abrasion, chemical injury, microbial invasion, and other insults associated with the passage of swallowed food, liquids, and gastric refluxate. A complex array of defense mechanisms, including structural components, secretory products, cellular processes, and immune responses, collectively contribute to the maintenance of mucosal integrity and homeostasis within the esophagus.

Structural Components:

1. **Stratified Squamous Epithelium:** The esophageal mucosa is lined by nonkeratinized stratified squamous epithelium, which provides a protective barrier against mechanical abrasion and chemical injury. Tight junctions between epithelial cells prevent the penetration of luminal contents and maintain mucosal integrity.
2. **Mucus Layer:** Surface epithelial cells and submucosal glands secrete mucus, a viscoelastic gel composed of glycoproteins and water, which coats the luminal surface of the esophagus and provides lubrication to facilitate the passage of swallowed material. Mucus also acts as a physical barrier that traps particulate matter and pathogens, preventing direct contact with the underlying epithelium.
3. **Epithelial Turnover:** The esophageal epithelium undergoes continuous renewal through a process of cellular proliferation, migration, and differentiation, which serves to replace damaged or sloughed cells and maintain mucosal integrity. Rapid turnover of epithelial cells ensures efficient repair of superficial injuries and preservation of barrier function.

Secretory Products:

1. **Bicarbonate (HCO3-):** Surface epithelial cells and submucosal glands secrete bicarbonate-rich mucus, which helps neutralize luminal acid and buffer gastric refluxate, thereby reducing mucosal injury and inflammation. Bicarbonate secretion is stimulated by luminal acidification and mediated by chloride-bicarbonate exchange mechanisms.
2. **Prostaglandins:** Prostaglandins, particularly prostaglandin E2 (PGE2), are lipid-derived signaling molecules synthesized by surface epithelial cells and submucosal glands in response to mucosal injury and inflammation. They exert cytoprotective effects by promoting mucus secretion, vasodilation, and epithelial cell proliferation, while inhibiting gastric acid secretion and leukocyte activation.
3. **Antimicrobial Peptides:** The esophageal mucosa produces various antimicrobial peptides, including defensins, cathelicidins, and lysozyme, which possess broad-spectrum antimicrobial activity against bacteria, fungi, and viruses. These peptides help maintain microbial homeostasis within the esophageal lumen and prevent pathogen colonization and invasion.

Cellular Processes:

1. **Tight Junctions:** Intercellular tight junctions between adjacent epithelial cells form a semipermeable barrier that regulates paracellular transport of ions, solutes, and water across the epithelium. Tight junction proteins, such as occludins, claudins, and zonula occludens, control barrier permeability and prevent the diffusion of luminal antigens and pathogens into the underlying tissues.
2. **Desmosomes:** Desmosomal junctions provide

mechanical stability and cohesion between adjacent epithelial cells, anchoring them to the basement membrane and resisting shearing forces associated with luminal transit and peristaltic contractions. Desmosomal proteins, including desmogleins and desmocollins, maintain intercellular adhesion and tissue integrity.
3. **Epithelial Repair:** Surface epithelial cells possess regenerative capacity and undergo rapid proliferation in response to mucosal injury or inflammation. Enhanced epithelial migration and differentiation facilitate re-epithelialization of denuded areas and restoration of barrier function following injury.

Immune Responses:

1. **Innate Immunity:** The esophageal mucosa is equipped with innate immune cells, including macrophages, dendritic cells, and intraepithelial lymphocytes, which survey the luminal environment for potential pathogens and initiate immune responses. Toll-like receptors (TLRs) recognize microbial antigens and activate inflammatory signaling pathways, leading to cytokine production and recruitment of effector cells.
2. **Mucosal Immunoglobulins:** Secretory immunoglobulin A (IgA) antibodies are produced by plasma cells within the esophageal lamina propria and mucosal-associated lymphoid tissue (MALT) in response to luminal antigens and pathogens. IgA antibodies bind to microbial antigens and toxins, neutralizing their virulence and preventing adherence to epithelial surfaces.
3. **Inflammatory Mediators:** Proinflammatory cytokines, such as interleukin-1 (IL-1), interleukin-6 (IL-6), and tumor necrosis factor-alpha (TNF-α), are produced by resident immune cells and activated

epithelial cells in response to mucosal injury, infection, or inflammation. These mediators promote vasodilation, leukocyte recruitment, and tissue repair processes within the esophageal mucosa.

In summary, the esophageal mucosal barrier encompasses a multifaceted network of structural components, secretory products, cellular processes, and immune responses that collectively protect against mechanical, chemical, and microbial insults associated with luminal transit and gastric reflux. Preservation of mucosal integrity and homeostasis is essential for maintaining esophageal health and preventing the development of inflammatory disorders such as esophagitis. Understanding the mucosal defense mechanisms of the esophagus provides insights into its role in host defense, barrier function, and disease pathogenesis.

Peristalsis and Esophageal Motility

Peristalsis and esophageal motility are fundamental physiological processes that facilitate the transport of swallowed food and liquids from the pharynx to the stomach. Coordinated contraction and relaxation of esophageal smooth muscle, orchestrated by neural reflexes and hormonal signals, ensure efficient propulsion of boluses through the esophagus while maintaining barrier integrity and preventing reflux of gastric contents.

Neural Control of Esophageal Motility:

1. **Enteric Nervous System:** The enteric nervous system (ENS), also known as the "brain in the gut,"

consists of a complex network of ganglia and nerve fibers embedded within the wall of the esophagus. The ENS regulates esophageal motility autonomously, coordinating peristalsis and sphincter function in response to local sensory inputs and motor commands.

2. **Vagal Innervation:** Parasympathetic innervation of the esophagus is primarily provided by the vagus nerve (cranial nerve X), which supplies preganglionic fibers to the myenteric (Auerbach's) plexus and submucosal (Meissner's) plexus of the ENS. Vagal efferent fibers release acetylcholine (ACh) at synapses with postganglionic neurons, smooth muscle cells, and interstitial cells of Cajal (ICC), promoting muscle contraction and sphincter relaxation.

3. **Cholinergic Transmission:** Acetylcholine (ACh) acts as the primary neurotransmitter mediating excitatory cholinergic transmission within the esophageal wall. Released from vagal efferent terminals and enteric neurons, ACh binds to muscarinic receptors on smooth muscle cells, initiating depolarization and calcium influx, which triggers contraction and propagates peristalsis.

4. **Inhibitory Neurons:** In addition to excitatory cholinergic neurons, the ENS contains inhibitory motor neurons that release nitric oxide (NO) and vasoactive intestinal peptide (VIP). These inhibitory neurotransmitters hyperpolarize smooth muscle cells, decrease intracellular calcium levels, and promote muscle relaxation, facilitating the coordinated relaxation of the LES and inhibition of non-propulsive contractions.

Mechanism of Esophageal Peristalsis:

1. **Swallowing Reflex:** The initiation of esophageal

peristalsis is triggered by the act of swallowing (deglutition), which involves a coordinated sequence of voluntary and involuntary muscle contractions in the oral cavity, pharynx, and esophagus. The swallowing reflex is divided into three phases: oral (voluntary), pharyngeal (involuntary), and esophageal (involuntary).
2. **Primary Peristalsis:** Primary peristalsis refers to the sequential contraction of esophageal smooth muscle that propels a swallowed bolus from the pharynx to the stomach. It is initiated by the pharyngeal phase of swallowing and propagated along the entire length of the esophagus via a wave of coordinated muscle contraction and relaxation.
3. **Peristaltic Wave:** The peristaltic wave consists of two components: a leading contraction (or contraction ring) that advances the bolus distally and a trailing relaxation (or inhibition zone) that follows behind, allowing for bolus transit and preventing retrograde flow of luminal contents. The wave of contraction is initiated by localized depolarization of smooth muscle cells and spreads rapidly along the esophageal wall via intercellular electrical coupling and gap junctions.
4. **Neurohumoral Regulation:** Peristalsis is modulated by neural reflexes, hormonal signals, and local factors within the esophageal wall. Distension of the esophageal lumen by a swallowed bolus activates sensory receptors (mechanoreceptors and stretch receptors) in the mucosa and muscularis propria, which transmit signals to the central nervous system (CNS) via vagal afferent fibers. Efferent signals from the CNS then trigger motor responses in the ENS, coordinating muscle contraction and relaxation to propel the bolus distally.

Secondary Peristalsis and Receptive Relaxation:

1. **Secondary Peristalsis:** Secondary peristalsis refers to the reflexive contraction of esophageal smooth muscle in response to esophageal distension, mucosal irritation, or the presence of residual material within the esophagus. It serves to clear retained boluses, refluxed gastric contents, or luminal debris from the esophageal lumen, ensuring efficient transit and clearance.
2. **Receptive Relaxation:** Receptive relaxation is a coordinated reflex response that occurs in the proximal esophagus and LES in anticipation of swallowing. It involves transient relaxation of the LES and inhibition of non-propulsive contractions in the proximal esophagus, allowing for unimpeded passage of swallowed material into the stomach without generating intraluminal pressure gradients or resistance.

Clinical Implications:

1. **Esophageal Dysmotility Disorders:** Disorders of esophageal motility, such as achalasia, diffuse esophageal spasm (DES), and ineffective esophageal motility (IEM), can impair the coordinated propulsion of swallowed boluses and disrupt the function of the LES, leading to dysphagia, regurgitation, chest pain, and reflux symptoms. Diagnosis of esophageal dysmotility disorders often involves esophageal manometry, impedance studies, and functional imaging techniques.
2. **Gastroesophageal Reflux Disease (GERD):** Impaired esophageal peristalsis and LES dysfunction are key pathophysiological mechanisms underlying GERD,

allowing for retrograde flow of gastric contents into the esophagus and promoting mucosal injury and inflammation. Treatment of GERD may involve lifestyle modifications, pharmacotherapy (e.g., proton pump inhibitors), and surgical interventions (e.g., fundoplication) aimed at restoring barrier function and preventing reflux events.
3. **Esophageal Transit Disorders:** Disorders affecting esophageal motility and transit, such as scleroderma, eosinophilic esophagitis (EoE), and systemic sclerosis, can result in dysphagia, food impaction, and bolus retention due to impaired peristalsis, strictures, or mucosal inflammation. Management of esophageal transit disorders may require dietary modifications, endoscopic dilation, and immunosuppressive therapy targeting underlying inflammatory processes.

In summary, peristalsis and esophageal motility are essential physiological processes that facilitate the transport of swallowed material through the esophagus and into the stomach. Coordinated neural reflexes, hormonal signals, and local factors regulate muscle contraction and relaxation, ensuring efficient propulsion of boluses while maintaining barrier integrity and preventing reflux of gastric contents. Dysfunction of esophageal motility can lead to a range of clinical symptoms and disorders, highlighting the importance of understanding the mechanisms underlying esophageal peristalsis and motility regulation.

Neurological Control of Esophageal Function

The neurological control of esophageal function is a

complex interplay between central and peripheral nervous system components, involving intricate neural circuits, neurotransmitters, and receptors that regulate swallowing, peristalsis, sphincter tone, and sensory perception within the esophagus. Understanding the neuroanatomy and neurophysiology underlying esophageal function provides insights into the mechanisms of normal physiology and the pathophysiology of neurogenic disorders affecting esophageal motility.

Neural Anatomy of the Esophagus:

1. **Vagal Innervation:** Parasympathetic innervation of the esophagus is primarily supplied by the vagus nerve (cranial nerve X), which originates from the medulla oblongata and contains both afferent (sensory) and efferent (motor) fibers. The vagus nerve gives rise to branches that form the esophageal plexus, including the myenteric (Auerbach's) plexus and submucosal (Meissner's) plexus, which innervate the muscularis propria and mucosa, respectively.
2. **Enteric Nervous System (ENS):** The ENS, often referred to as the "second brain," is a complex network of ganglia and nerve fibers located within the wall of the esophagus. It consists of two main plexuses: the myenteric plexus, located between the longitudinal and circular muscle layers, and the submucosal plexus, situated within the submucosal layer. The ENS integrates sensory input, coordinates motor output, and regulates esophageal motility independently of central nervous system (CNS) input.
3. **Extrinsic Innervation:** In addition to vagal innervation, the esophagus receives sympathetic innervation from the thoracic splanchnic nerves, which originate from the sympathetic chain ganglia in the thoracic spinal cord. Sympathetic fibers modulate

vascular tone, glandular secretion, and smooth muscle contraction within the esophageal wall, often in conjunction with parasympathetic control.

Neurotransmitters and Receptors:

1. **Acetylcholine (ACh):** ACh is the primary neurotransmitter released by vagal efferent (motor) neurons and enteric neurons within the esophageal wall. It acts on muscarinic receptors located on smooth muscle cells, interstitial cells of Cajal (ICC), and enteric neurons to promote smooth muscle contraction, sphincter relaxation, and neurotransmission.
2. **Nitric Oxide (NO):** NO is a potent inhibitory neurotransmitter released by inhibitory motor neurons within the ENS. It diffuses across cell membranes and activates soluble guanylate cyclase (sGC) in smooth muscle cells, leading to increased levels of cyclic guanosine monophosphate (cGMP) and smooth muscle relaxation. NO-mediated relaxation of the lower esophageal sphincter (LES) and inhibitory regulation of peristalsis contribute to esophageal motor function and sphincter control.
3. **Vasoactive Intestinal Peptide (VIP):** VIP is a neurotransmitter and neuropeptide released by inhibitory motor neurons within the ENS. It acts on smooth muscle cells and secretory glands to promote relaxation and inhibit contraction, modulating esophageal motility and secretion. VIP-mediated effects are mediated by cyclic adenosine monophosphate (cAMP) signaling pathways and receptor activation.
4. **Substance P:** Substance P is a neuropeptide released by sensory (afferent) neurons within the esophageal mucosa in response to mechanical, chemical, or

thermal stimuli. It acts as a neurotransmitter and nociceptive mediator, transmitting sensory signals related to esophageal distension, pain, and reflexive responses. Substance P receptors are localized on both sensory neurons and interneurons within the ENS, modulating sensory transmission and neural excitability.

Neural Reflexes and Motor Patterns:

1. **Swallowing Reflex:** The swallowing reflex is initiated by sensory receptors in the oral cavity and pharynx, which transmit signals to the brainstem swallowing center located in the medulla oblongata. Efferent signals from the swallowing center activate motor neurons in the nucleus ambiguus and dorsal motor nucleus of the vagus, initiating a coordinated sequence of muscle contractions and relaxations in the oral, pharyngeal, and esophageal musculature.
2. **Peristaltic Reflex:** The peristaltic reflex is a localized reflex arc within the esophageal wall, involving sensory receptors, interneurons, and motor neurons of the ENS. Distension of the esophageal lumen by a swallowed bolus activates mechanoreceptors and stretch receptors, which transmit signals to interneurons in the myenteric plexus. Excitatory motor neurons release ACh and other neurotransmitters, stimulating smooth muscle contraction and propagating a peristaltic wave distally along the esophagus.
3. **Receptive Relaxation:** Receptive relaxation is a vagally mediated reflex response that occurs in the proximal esophagus and LES in anticipation of swallowing. Sensory input from the esophageal mucosa activates inhibitory motor neurons in the myenteric plexus, which release NO and VIP to induce

transient relaxation of the LES and inhibition of non-propulsive contractions, facilitating bolus transit into the stomach.

Clinical Implications:

1. **Neurogenic Dysphagia:** Neurological disorders affecting central or peripheral components of the swallowing reflex, such as stroke, Parkinson's disease, multiple sclerosis, or neuropathies, can result in neurogenic dysphagia characterized by impaired initiation, coordination, or propulsion of swallowed boluses. Management of neurogenic dysphagia may involve swallowing rehabilitation, dietary modifications, and targeted therapies to address underlying neurological deficits.

2. **Esophageal Motility Disorders:** Dysfunction of esophageal motor function, secondary to neuromuscular disorders, ENS abnormalities, or neurotransmitter imbalances, can lead to esophageal motility disorders such as achalasia, diffuse esophageal spasm (DES), or hypertensive peristalsis. Diagnosis of esophageal motility disorders often requires esophageal manometry, impedance studies, and functional imaging techniques to assess peristaltic coordination, LES tone, and bolus transit.

3. **Neurogenic Reflux:** Impaired esophageal clearance, LES dysfunction, or alterations in sensory perception due to neurological deficits can predispose individuals to gastroesophageal reflux disease (GERD) and reflux-related complications. Management of neurogenic reflux may involve lifestyle modifications, pharmacotherapy (e.g., proton pump inhibitors), and surgical interventions (e.g., fundoplication) to reduce acid reflux and improve esophageal function.

In summary, the neurological control of esophageal function involves intricate neural circuits, neurotransmitters, and receptors that regulate swallowing, peristalsis, sphincter tone, and sensory perception within the esophagus. Central and peripheral nervous system components coordinate esophageal motility and sensory responses, ensuring efficient bolus transit, barrier integrity, and reflexive control of esophageal function. Dysfunction of the neural control mechanisms can lead to a range of clinical symptoms and disorders affecting esophageal motility and function, highlighting the importance of understanding the neuroanatomy and neurophysiology underlying esophageal function.

CHAPTER 3: GASTROESOPHAGEAL REFLUX DISEASE (GERD) AND ESOPHAGITIS

Introduction

Gastroesophageal reflux disease (GERD) and esophagitis are closely intertwined entities, with GERD being one of the primary causes of esophagitis. GERD is characterized by the reflux of gastric contents, including acid, bile salts, and pepsin, into the esophagus, leading to mucosal injury, inflammation, and symptomatic manifestations. Esophagitis refers to inflammation of the esophageal mucosa, which can result from various etiologies, with GERD being the most common cause. Understanding the relationship between GERD and esophagitis is crucial for accurate diagnosis, appropriate management, and prevention of complications associated with these conditions.

Pathophysiology of GERD and Esophagitis:

1. **Gastroesophageal Reflux:** GERD arises from the inappropriate reflux of gastric contents into the esophagus due to dysfunction of the lower esophageal sphincter (LES) or impaired esophageal clearance mechanisms. Factors contributing to reflux include transient relaxation of the LES, decreased LES pressure, hiatal hernia, delayed gastric emptying, and increased intra-abdominal pressure. Refluxed gastric contents contain acid, bile salts, pepsin, and other digestive enzymes, which can injure the esophageal mucosa and trigger inflammatory responses.
2. **Esophageal Mucosal Injury:** Prolonged exposure of the esophageal mucosa to acidic and enzymatic components of gastric refluxate leads to mucosal injury and inflammation. Acidic pH disrupts the protective mucosal barrier, impairs epithelial cell integrity, and activates inflammatory pathways, resulting in mucosal erosions, ulcerations, and microabscess formation. Bile salts and pepsin further exacerbate mucosal damage by inducing cytotoxic effects, oxidative stress, and proteolytic degradation of proteins.
3. **Inflammatory Responses:** Esophageal mucosal injury triggers inflammatory responses characterized by the infiltration of inflammatory cells, release of proinflammatory cytokines, and activation of immune mediators within the esophageal wall. Neutrophils, eosinophils, lymphocytes, and mast cells accumulate in the submucosa and lamina propria, releasing cytokines such as interleukin-1 (IL-1), interleukin-6 (IL-6), tumor necrosis factor-alpha (TNF-α), and transforming growth factor-beta (TGF-β). These cytokines mediate tissue damage, fibroblast

activation, collagen deposition, and remodeling processes that contribute to esophageal inflammation and fibrosis.

Clinical Manifestations of GERD and Esophagitis:

1. **Heartburn:** Heartburn, characterized by a burning sensation in the retrosternal or epigastric region, is the hallmark symptom of GERD and esophagitis. It typically worsens after meals, when lying down, or during nocturnal periods, reflecting the exacerbation of reflux events and mucosal irritation. Heartburn may be accompanied by regurgitation of acidic or bitter-tasting fluid into the mouth, known as acid regurgitation.
2. **Dysphagia:** Dysphagia, or difficulty swallowing, can occur in patients with GERD and esophagitis due to esophageal mucosal injury, strictures, or motility disturbances. Dysphagia may present as a sensation of food sticking or catching in the throat, particularly with solid foods, and may be associated with pain, discomfort, or a feeling of fullness in the chest.
3. **Odynophagia:** Odynophagia, or painful swallowing, is a common symptom of esophagitis resulting from mucosal erosions, ulcerations, or inflammation. Patients may experience sharp, stabbing pain in the chest or throat upon swallowing, which may be exacerbated by acidic or spicy foods, hot liquids, or vigorous swallowing.
4. **Regurgitation:** Regurgitation refers to the passive reflux of gastric contents into the esophagus or oral cavity, resulting in the sensation of fluid or food returning from the stomach. Regurgitation may be accompanied by a sour or bitter taste in the mouth, halitosis (bad breath), or aspiration of gastric contents into the respiratory tract, leading to coughing,

wheezing, or respiratory symptoms.

Diagnostic Evaluation:

1. **Upper Endoscopy:** Upper endoscopy, or esophagogastroduodenoscopy (EGD), is the gold standard diagnostic modality for evaluating esophageal mucosal injury and inflammation in patients with suspected GERD or esophagitis. EGD allows for direct visualization of the esophageal mucosa, assessment of mucosal integrity, identification of erosions or ulcers, and sampling of tissue specimens for histological examination.
2. **Esophageal pH Monitoring:** Esophageal pH monitoring is a valuable diagnostic tool for quantifying acid reflux episodes and assessing esophageal acid exposure in patients with GERD. Ambulatory pH monitoring using a pH probe placed within the distal esophagus allows for continuous monitoring of intraesophageal pH levels over a 24-hour period, providing objective data on reflux frequency, duration, and pH parameters.
3. **Esophageal Manometry:** Esophageal manometry evaluates esophageal motility and LES function by measuring intraluminal pressures and peristaltic wave characteristics along the length of the esophagus. Manometric findings can help identify motility disorders, such as achalasia or ineffective esophageal motility, which may predispose patients to reflux events and esophageal inflammation.

Management Strategies:

1. **Lifestyle Modifications:** Lifestyle modifications are recommended as first-line therapy for GERD and esophagitis and include dietary changes, weight loss,

elevation of the head of the bed, avoidance of trigger foods (e.g., caffeine, alcohol, spicy foods), and cessation of smoking. These measures aim to reduce reflux events, alleviate symptoms, and promote esophageal healing.
2. **Pharmacotherapy:** Pharmacotherapy options for GERD and esophagitis include antacids, histamine H2-receptor antagonists (H2RAs), proton pump inhibitors (PPIs), prokinetic agents, and mucosal protectants. PPIs are the most effective agents for suppressing gastric acid secretion and healing esophageal mucosal injury, achieving symptom relief in the majority of patients.
3. **Endoscopic Therapy:** Endoscopic therapy may be considered for patients with refractory GERD symptoms or complications such as erosive esophagitis, strictures, or Barrett's esophagus. Endoscopic interventions, such as radiofrequency ablation (RFA), endoscopic mucosal resection (EMR), or endoscopic suturing, aim to improve LES function, reduce reflux burden, and prevent disease progression.

Complications and Prognosis:

1. **Strictures:** Chronic inflammation and fibrosis of the esophageal mucosa can lead to the formation of esophageal strictures, or narrowing of the esophageal lumen, which may cause dysphagia, food impaction, or obstructive symptoms. Strictures may require endoscopic dilation or surgical intervention to alleviate symptoms and restore luminal patency.
2. **Barrett's Esophagus:** Barrett's esophagus is a premalignant condition characterized by the replacement of normal squamous epithelium with specialized intestinal metaplasia in response to chronic gastroesophageal reflux. Patients with

Barrett's esophagus are at increased risk of developing esophageal adenocarcinoma, highlighting the importance of surveillance endoscopy and dysplasia detection.

3. **Adenocarcinoma:** Chronic inflammation and epithelial damage associated with GERD and esophagitis can predispose patients to the development of esophageal adenocarcinoma, a malignant neoplasm arising from Barrett's esophagus or dysplastic epithelium. Early detection, surveillance, and aggressive management of GERD and esophagitis are essential for reducing the risk of adenocarcinoma progression and improving patient outcomes.

In summary, GERD and esophagitis are closely linked conditions characterized by the reflux of gastric contents into the esophagus, leading to mucosal injury, inflammation, and symptomatic manifestations. Understanding the pathophysiology, clinical manifestations, diagnostic evaluation, and management strategies of GERD and esophagitis is essential for accurate diagnosis, appropriate treatment, and prevention of complications associated with these conditions. Early recognition and intervention are crucial for optimizing patient outcomes and reducing the risk of long-term complications such as strictures, Barrett's esophagus, and esophageal adenocarcinoma.

Pathogenesis of GERD-Associated Esophagitis

Gastroesophageal reflux disease (GERD)-associated esophagitis develops as a result of the complex interplay between several pathophysiological factors, including dysfunction of the lower esophageal sphincter (LES), impaired esophageal clearance mechanisms, mucosal susceptibility to injury, and inflammatory responses to refluxed gastric contents. Understanding the pathogenesis of GERD-associated esophagitis is crucial for elucidating the mechanisms underlying mucosal damage and inflammation, guiding diagnostic evaluation, and informing therapeutic interventions aimed at preventing mucosal injury and symptom exacerbation.

Lower Esophageal Sphincter Dysfunction:

1. **Transient Relaxation of LES:** The primary mechanism underlying GERD pathogenesis involves transient relaxation of the lower esophageal sphincter (LES), a specialized ring of smooth muscle located at the gastroesophageal junction (GEJ) that serves as a physiological barrier to reflux. Transient LES relaxation (TLESR) occurs in response to various stimuli, including gastric distension, meal ingestion, esophageal distension, and central nervous system (CNS) activation, leading to temporary relaxation of the sphincter and opening of the GEJ.

2. **Decreased LES Pressure:** In addition to TLESR, GERD may be associated with a decrease in basal LES pressure, predisposing individuals to spontaneous reflux episodes and impaired barrier function. Factors contributing to decreased LES pressure include genetic predisposition, obesity, hiatal hernia, tobacco smoking, and certain medications (e.g., calcium channel blockers, nitrates), which can disrupt the normal neuromuscular control of LES tone and sphincter function.

Impaired Esophageal Clearance Mechanisms:

1. **Delayed Gastric Emptying:** Delayed gastric emptying,

or gastroparesis, can promote GERD by prolonging the retention of gastric contents within the stomach and increasing the likelihood of refluxate reaching the esophagus. Conditions associated with delayed gastric emptying, such as diabetes mellitus, neuropathic disorders, and gastric dysmotility syndromes, may exacerbate GERD symptoms and contribute to esophageal mucosal injury.

2. **Hiatal Hernia:** Hiatal hernia, characterized by the protrusion of the gastric cardia above the diaphragmatic hiatus into the thoracic cavity, is a common anatomical abnormality associated with GERD. Hiatal hernia disrupts the integrity of the GEJ and impairs LES function, allowing for easier passage of gastric contents into the esophagus and increasing the risk of reflux-induced esophagitis.

Mucosal Susceptibility to Injury:

1. **Decreased Mucosal Resistance:** The esophageal mucosa is normally protected by a layer of mucus, bicarbonate secretion, epithelial cell turnover, and reparative mechanisms that serve to maintain mucosal integrity and resist injury. However, in individuals with GERD, factors such as chronic acid exposure, bile reflux, pepsin activity, and impaired mucosal defense mechanisms can compromise mucosal resistance and increase susceptibility to injury.

2. **Acid and Pepsin Exposure:** Acidic refluxate from the stomach contains hydrochloric acid (HCl), which has a low pH and can directly injure the esophageal mucosa through chemical burns, denaturation of proteins, and disruption of intercellular junctions. Additionally, pepsin, a proteolytic enzyme produced by gastric chief cells, is activated by acidic pH and can degrade

mucosal proteins, exacerbating mucosal injury and inflammation in GERD-associated esophagitis.

Inflammatory Responses:

1. **Neutrophil Infiltration:** Inflammatory responses to mucosal injury in GERD-associated esophagitis are characterized by the infiltration of inflammatory cells, predominantly neutrophils, into the esophageal mucosa and submucosa. Neutrophil recruitment is mediated by chemotactic factors released by injured epithelial cells, such as interleukin-8 (IL-8), which promote leukocyte migration and activation at sites of tissue damage.

2. **Cytokine Release:** In response to mucosal injury and inflammatory stimuli, resident immune cells and epithelial cells produce proinflammatory cytokines, including interleukin-1 (IL-1), interleukin-6 (IL-6), tumor necrosis factor-alpha (TNF-α), and interferon-gamma (IFN-γ). These cytokines orchestrate inflammatory cascades, amplify immune responses, and perpetuate tissue damage and repair processes within the esophageal mucosa.

3. **Oxidative Stress:** Reactive oxygen species (ROS) generated during GERD-associated reflux events contribute to oxidative stress and oxidative damage within the esophageal mucosa, leading to lipid peroxidation, protein oxidation, DNA damage, and mitochondrial dysfunction. Oxidative stress exacerbates mucosal injury, promotes inflammation, and impairs tissue repair mechanisms, further compromising mucosal integrity and barrier function.

Clinical Implications and Management Strategies:

1. **Proton Pump Inhibitors (PPIs):** Proton pump

inhibitors (PPIs) are the mainstay of pharmacological therapy for GERD-associated esophagitis, exerting potent acid-suppressive effects by inhibiting the H+/K+-ATPase pump in gastric parietal cells. PPIs reduce gastric acid secretion, alleviate symptoms, promote esophageal healing, and prevent recurrence of mucosal injury in patients with GERD.

2. **Mucosal Protectants:** Mucosal protectants, such as alginate-based formulations, sucralfate, and prostaglandin analogs, may be used adjunctively with PPIs to enhance mucosal defense mechanisms, promote mucosal healing, and provide symptomatic relief in patients with GERD-associated esophagitis.

3. **Lifestyle Modifications:** Lifestyle modifications, including dietary changes, weight loss, elevation of the head of the bed, avoidance of trigger foods (e.g., caffeine, alcohol, spicy foods), and cessation of tobacco smoking, are recommended as adjunctive measures to reduce reflux symptoms, minimize mucosal injury, and optimize treatment outcomes in patients with GERD.

In summary, the pathogenesis of GERD-associated esophagitis involves a multifactorial interplay between LES dysfunction, impaired esophageal clearance mechanisms, mucosal susceptibility to injury, and inflammatory responses to refluxed gastric contents. Understanding the underlying mechanisms of mucosal damage and inflammation informs diagnostic evaluation and therapeutic interventions aimed at preventing mucosal injury, alleviating symptoms, and optimizing patient outcomes in GERD-associated esophagitis. Early recognition and management of GERD are essential for preventing progression to esophageal complications such as strictures, Barrett's esophagus, and esophageal adenocarcinoma.

Clinical Manifestations and Diagnostic Criteria

Clinical manifestations and diagnostic criteria play a pivotal role in the assessment and management of gastroesophageal reflux disease (GERD) and esophagitis. Recognizing the diverse array of symptoms and employing appropriate diagnostic tools are essential for accurate diagnosis, tailored treatment strategies, and prevention of complications associated with these conditions.

Clinical Manifestations:

1. **Heartburn:** Heartburn, a burning sensation behind the breastbone or sternum, is the hallmark symptom of GERD and esophagitis. It typically occurs after meals or when lying down and may worsen with bending over or lifting. Heartburn is often described as a retrosternal discomfort that may radiate to the neck, throat, or back, mimicking symptoms of cardiac origin.
2. **Regurgitation:** Regurgitation refers to the reflux of gastric contents into the esophagus or oral cavity, leading to the sensation of fluid or food coming back up. Patients may experience a sour or bitter taste in the mouth, acidic regurgitation, or the feeling of a lump or obstruction in the throat. Regurgitation may occur spontaneously or be triggered by bending, lying down, or eating large meals.
3. **Dysphagia:** Dysphagia, or difficulty swallowing, is a common symptom of esophagitis resulting from mucosal inflammation, strictures, or motility

disturbances. Patients may experience pain or discomfort upon swallowing, sensation of food sticking in the throat or chest, or difficulty swallowing solids or liquids. Dysphagia may be intermittent or progressive and may be associated with weight loss or aspiration.

4. **Odynophagia:** Odynophagia, or painful swallowing, may accompany esophagitis and is characterized by sharp, stabbing pain in the chest or throat upon swallowing. Patients may experience localized pain or discomfort that worsens with ingestion of hot, spicy, or acidic foods, as well as with rapid swallowing or vigorous coughing. Odynophagia may indicate mucosal erosions, ulcerations, or inflammation.

5. **Non-cardiac Chest Pain:** Non-cardiac chest pain, or atypical chest pain unrelated to cardiac pathology, is a common manifestation of GERD and esophagitis. Patients may describe a burning, squeezing, or pressure-like sensation in the chest that is not relieved by nitroglycerin or antacids. Non-cardiac chest pain may be exacerbated by eating, lying down, or bending over and may be associated with anxiety or stress.

6. **Respiratory Symptoms:** GERD-associated reflux events can trigger respiratory symptoms, such as coughing, wheezing, hoarseness, or asthma exacerbations, due to aspiration of gastric contents into the airways. Microaspiration of acidic or non-acidic refluxate can irritate the respiratory mucosa, induce bronchoconstriction, or stimulate cough receptors, leading to respiratory symptoms and exacerbations.

Diagnostic Criteria:

1. **Symptom Assessment:** Diagnosis of GERD and esophagitis begins with a thorough clinical evaluation

of presenting symptoms, including frequency, duration, severity, triggers, and response to treatment. Symptom assessment, using standardized questionnaires such as the Gastroesophageal Reflux Disease Questionnaire (GERD-Q) or Reflux Symptom Index (RSI), helps quantify symptom severity and monitor treatment response over time.
2. **Upper Endoscopy:** Upper endoscopy, or esophagogastroduodenoscopy (EGD), is the gold standard diagnostic modality for evaluating esophageal mucosal injury and inflammation in patients with suspected GERD or esophagitis. EGD allows for direct visualization of the esophageal mucosa, assessment of mucosal integrity, identification of erosions or ulcers, and sampling of tissue specimens for histological examination.
3. **Endoscopic Findings:** Endoscopic findings suggestive of esophagitis include erythema, edema, erosions, ulcerations, friability, or strictures of the esophageal mucosa. The Los Angeles classification system grades the severity of esophagitis based on the extent and severity of mucosal damage, ranging from mild (grade A) to severe (grade D) esophagitis.
4. **Biopsy and Histopathology:** Tissue biopsy specimens obtained during upper endoscopy can provide valuable histological information regarding the nature and severity of esophageal mucosal inflammation, as well as the presence of eosinophilic infiltrates, neutrophilic microabscesses, or Barrett's esophagus. Histological evaluation helps confirm the diagnosis of esophagitis and identify underlying etiologies, such as eosinophilic esophagitis or infectious causes.
5. **Esophageal pH Monitoring:** Esophageal pH monitoring is a valuable diagnostic tool for quantifying acid reflux episodes and assessing

esophageal acid exposure in patients with GERD. Ambulatory pH monitoring using a pH probe placed within the distal esophagus allows for continuous monitoring of intraesophageal pH levels over a 24-hour period, providing objective data on reflux frequency, duration, and pH parameters.
6. **Esophageal Manometry:** Esophageal manometry evaluates esophageal motility and LES function by measuring intraluminal pressures and peristaltic wave characteristics along the length of the esophagus. Manometric findings can help identify motility disorders, such as achalasia or ineffective esophageal motility, which may predispose patients to reflux events and esophageal inflammation.

Clinical Implications:

1. **Diagnostic Algorithm:** A systematic approach to the diagnosis of GERD and esophagitis involves a combination of clinical assessment, endoscopic evaluation, and ancillary testing to establish the diagnosis, characterize the severity of mucosal injury, and identify potential complications. Integration of symptom assessment, endoscopic findings, and objective testing helps guide treatment decisions and monitor treatment response over time.
2. **Treatment Tailoring:** Tailoring treatment strategies to individual patient characteristics, symptom severity, and diagnostic findings is essential for optimizing therapeutic outcomes and minimizing treatment-related adverse effects. Patient education, lifestyle modifications, pharmacotherapy, and procedural interventions should be tailored to address specific symptoms, comorbidities, and underlying pathophysiological mechanisms of GERD and esophagitis.

3. **Monitoring and Surveillance:** Long-term management of GERD and esophagitis requires regular monitoring of symptoms, endoscopic findings, and treatment response to assess disease progression, treatment efficacy, and adherence to therapy. Surveillance endoscopy may be indicated in patients with Barrett's esophagus or high-grade dysplasia to detect early neoplastic changes and prevent progression to esophageal adenocarcinoma.

In summary, clinical manifestations and diagnostic criteria are integral components of the evaluation and management of GERD and esophagitis. Recognizing the diverse array of symptoms, employing appropriate diagnostic modalities, and tailoring treatment strategies to individual patient characteristics are essential for accurate

Complications of GERD-Induced Esophagitis

Gastroesophageal reflux disease (GERD) can lead to a spectrum of complications, ranging from mucosal injury and inflammation to structural changes and malignant transformation of the esophagus. Understanding the potential complications associated with GERD-induced esophagitis is crucial for risk stratification, early detection, and targeted intervention to prevent long-term sequelae and improve patient outcomes.

1. Esophageal Strictures:

Esophageal strictures are characterized by the narrowing of the esophageal lumen due to fibrotic scarring and collagen deposition within the esophageal wall. Prolonged exposure to acidic refluxate in GERD-induced esophagitis can lead to chronic inflammation, ulceration, and healing by fibrosis, resulting in the formation of strictures. Patients with esophageal strictures may experience dysphagia, odynophagia, or food impaction, particularly with solid foods. Endoscopic dilation is the primary treatment modality for relieving symptoms and restoring luminal patency in patients with esophageal strictures.

2. Barrett's Esophagus:

Barrett's esophagus is a premalignant condition characterized by the replacement of normal squamous epithelium with specialized intestinal metaplasia in response to chronic gastroesophageal reflux. Patients with Barrett's esophagus are at increased risk of developing esophageal adenocarcinoma, a lethal malignancy with poor prognosis. Endoscopic surveillance with biopsies is recommended for patients with Barrett's esophagus to detect dysplastic changes and early neoplastic lesions. Management strategies for Barrett's esophagus include acid suppression therapy, endoscopic ablation techniques (e.g., radiofrequency ablation), and surgical resection in select cases.

3. Esophageal Ulcerations:

Esophageal ulcerations are focal defects or erosions in the esophageal mucosa that result from prolonged exposure to gastric acid, bile salts, and pepsin in GERD-induced esophagitis. Ulcerations may present with chest pain, dysphagia, or hematemesis and can lead to complications such as bleeding, perforation, or stricturing if left untreated. Endoscopic evaluation with biopsy is essential for diagnosing and managing esophageal ulcerations, with treatment aimed at acid suppression, mucosal protection, and supportive care to promote healing.

4. Hemorrhage:

Hemorrhage from esophageal mucosal erosions or ulcerations can occur in severe cases of GERD-induced esophagitis, leading to hematemesis, melena, or hematochezia. Patients with underlying coagulopathy, peptic ulcer disease, or advanced liver disease may be at increased risk of hemorrhagic complications. Endoscopic hemostasis, including injection therapy, thermal coagulation, or hemostatic clipping, may be required to control bleeding and prevent recurrence. Intravenous proton pump inhibitors (PPIs) and blood transfusion support may be necessary in hemodynamically unstable patients.

5. Perforation:

Esophageal perforation, though rare, is a potentially life-threatening complication of GERD-induced esophagitis that can result from severe mucosal injury, ulceration, or iatrogenic trauma during endoscopic procedures. Perforation may manifest as chest pain, dyspnea, subcutaneous emphysema, or septic shock and requires prompt recognition and intervention to prevent mediastinitis, abscess formation, or sepsis. Surgical repair, drainage of mediastinal collections, and broad-spectrum antibiotics are essential for managing esophageal perforation and preventing complications.

6. Respiratory Complications:

GERD-associated reflux events can trigger respiratory complications, such as aspiration pneumonia, bronchospasm, or exacerbations of underlying lung disease, due to aspiration of gastric contents into the airways. Patients with chronic respiratory conditions, such as asthma, chronic obstructive pulmonary disease (COPD), or interstitial lung disease, may be particularly susceptible to respiratory complications of GERD. Management strategies include aggressive treatment of reflux symptoms, optimization of respiratory therapy, and avoidance of exacerbating factors.

7. Dental Erosion:

Chronic exposure to acidic refluxate in GERD-induced esophagitis can lead to dental erosion, characterized by loss of tooth enamel and increased susceptibility to dental caries, tooth sensitivity, or tooth discoloration. Dental erosion typically affects the posterior teeth and may be associated with oral symptoms such as xerostomia, halitosis, or oropharyngeal discomfort. Oral hygiene measures, fluoride supplementation, and dental interventions (e.g., dental sealants, restorations) are essential for preventing and managing dental erosion in patients with GERD.

8. Psychosocial Impact:

Chronic GERD and esophagitis can have a significant psychosocial impact on patients' quality of life, leading to anxiety, depression, social isolation, and impaired work productivity. Persistent reflux symptoms, medication side effects, dietary restrictions, and fear of complications may contribute to emotional distress and psychological morbidity in affected individuals. Multidisciplinary approaches, including cognitive-behavioral therapy, patient education, and social support networks, are essential for addressing the psychosocial needs of patients with GERD-induced esophagitis.

In summary, GERD-induced esophagitis can lead to a range of complications, including esophageal strictures, Barrett's esophagus, ulcerations, hemorrhage, perforation, respiratory complications, dental erosion, and psychosocial morbidity. Recognition of these complications, early intervention, and multidisciplinary management are essential for optimizing patient outcomes and reducing the risk of long-term sequelae associated with GERD. Patient education, lifestyle modifications, pharmacotherapy, endoscopic interventions, and surgical options may be employed to mitigate complications, alleviate symptoms, and improve quality of life in patients with GERD-induced esophagitis.

CHAPTER 4: INFECTIOUS ESOPHAGITIS

Overview of Infectious Agents

Infectious esophagitis is a condition characterized by inflammation of the esophageal mucosa caused by microbial pathogens. While gastroesophageal reflux disease (GERD) is the most common cause of esophagitis, infectious agents can also contribute to esophageal inflammation, particularly in immunocompromised individuals or those with underlying predisposing factors. Understanding the spectrum of infectious agents implicated in esophagitis is crucial for accurate diagnosis, appropriate management, and prevention of complications associated with these infections.

1. Candida Species:

Candida species, particularly Candida albicans, are the most common pathogens implicated in infectious esophagitis, accounting for the majority of cases in immunocompromised patients, such as those with HIV/AIDS, hematological malignancies, or solid organ transplantation. Candida esophagitis typically presents with odynophagia, dysphagia, or retrosternal pain and may be associated with oral thrush or oropharyngeal candidiasis. Diagnosis is established by endoscopic evaluation with biopsy, demonstrating fungal hyphae invading the esophageal mucosa, and confirmed by microbiological culture or histopathological examination.

2. Herpes Simplex Virus (HSV):

Herpes simplex virus (HSV) is another common infectious agent implicated in esophagitis, particularly in immunocompromised individuals or those with impaired cell-mediated immunity. HSV esophagitis typically presents with acute onset of odynophagia, dysphagia, fever, and malaise, often accompanied by orolabial or genital herpes lesions. Endoscopic findings may include shallow ulcers with raised borders and surrounding erythema or exudates. Diagnosis is confirmed by viral culture, polymerase chain reaction (PCR), or immunofluorescence staining of biopsy specimens obtained during endoscopy.

3. Cytomegalovirus (CMV):

Cytomegalovirus (CMV) esophagitis is predominantly observed in immunocompromised patients, such as those with HIV/AIDS, organ transplantation, or hematological malignancies, although it can also occur in immunocompetent individuals with severe systemic illness. CMV esophagitis typically presents with subacute or chronic symptoms, including odynophagia, dysphagia, weight loss, and fever. Endoscopic findings may include linear or serpiginous ulcers with raised borders and surrounding inflammation. Diagnosis is established by histopathological examination of biopsy specimens demonstrating characteristic cytoplasmic and nuclear inclusions consistent with CMV infection.

4. Fungal Infections (Non-Candida):

In addition to Candida species, other fungal pathogens, such as Aspergillus species, Cryptococcus neoformans, Histoplasma capsulatum, and Pneumocystis jirovecii, can cause esophageal infections, particularly in immunocompromised individuals with impaired cellular immunity or underlying pulmonary disease. Fungal esophagitis may present with nonspecific symptoms, including dysphagia, odynophagia, or retrosternal discomfort, and may be associated with systemic fungal infections or disseminated disease. Diagnosis is established by endoscopic evaluation with biopsy and confirmed by histopathological examination, fungal culture, or molecular testing.

5. Bacterial Infections:

Bacterial esophagitis is relatively rare but can occur secondary to esophageal instrumentation, chemical injury, or underlying motility disorders that predispose to bacterial overgrowth. Common bacterial pathogens implicated in esophagitis include Streptococcus species, Staphylococcus aureus, Escherichia coli, Klebsiella pneumoniae, and Mycobacterium tuberculosis. Bacterial esophagitis may present with symptoms such as odynophagia, dysphagia, fever, or chest pain and may be associated with underlying risk factors such as immunosuppression, esophageal strictures, or gastroesophageal reflux disease (GERD). Diagnosis is established by endoscopic evaluation with biopsy and confirmed by microbiological culture or histopathological examination of tissue specimens.

6. Parasitic Infections:

Parasitic esophagitis is rare but can occur in individuals with a history of travel to endemic regions or immunocompromised states. Parasitic pathogens implicated in esophagitis include Schistosoma species, Strongyloides stercoralis, Toxoplasma gondii, and Acanthamoeba species. Parasitic esophagitis may present with nonspecific symptoms such as dysphagia, odynophagia, or epigastric pain and may be associated with systemic parasitic infections or disseminated disease. Diagnosis is established by endoscopic evaluation with biopsy and confirmed by histopathological examination, serological testing, or molecular diagnostics.

Conclusion:

Infectious esophagitis encompasses a diverse spectrum of microbial pathogens that can cause inflammation of the esophageal mucosa, leading to a range of clinical manifestations and complications. Candida species, herpes simplex virus (HSV), cytomegalovirus (CMV), and other fungal, bacterial, and parasitic pathogens are implicated in infectious esophagitis, particularly in immunocompromised individuals or those with underlying predisposing factors. Prompt recognition, accurate diagnosis, and targeted antimicrobial therapy are essential for managing infectious esophagitis and preventing complications such as esophageal strictures, perforation, or dissemination of infection. Multidisciplinary approaches involving gastroenterologists, infectious disease specialists, and immunologists are often required for comprehensive evaluation and management of infectious esophagitis.

Common Pathogens and Opportunistic Infections

Infectious esophagitis encompasses a spectrum of microbial pathogens, including common pathogens and opportunistic infections, that can cause inflammation and mucosal injury in the esophagus. Understanding the etiology, clinical manifestations, and diagnostic approaches for these infectious agents is essential for accurate diagnosis and targeted management strategies.

1. Candida Species:

Candida species, particularly Candida albicans, are ubiquitous opportunistic fungal pathogens that commonly cause infectious esophagitis, particularly in immunocompromised individuals or those with predisposing factors such as diabetes mellitus, corticosteroid therapy, or HIV/AIDS. Candida esophagitis typically presents with symptoms such as odynophagia, dysphagia, or retrosternal discomfort and may be associated with oral thrush or oropharyngeal candidiasis. Endoscopic findings include white plaques, pseudomembranes, or erythematous mucosa, and diagnosis is confirmed by histopathological examination demonstrating fungal hyphae invading the esophageal mucosa.

2. Herpes Simplex Virus (HSV):

Herpes simplex virus (HSV) is a common viral pathogen implicated in infectious esophagitis, particularly in immunocompromised individuals or those with impaired cell-mediated immunity. HSV esophagitis typically presents with acute onset of symptoms, including severe odynophagia, dysphagia, fever, and malaise, often accompanied by orolabial or genital herpes lesions. Endoscopic findings may include shallow ulcers with raised borders and surrounding inflammation, and diagnosis is confirmed by viral culture, polymerase chain reaction (PCR), or immunofluorescence staining of biopsy specimens obtained during endoscopy.

3. Cytomegalovirus (CMV):

Cytomegalovirus (CMV) is another common viral pathogen associated with infectious esophagitis, particularly in immunocompromised individuals such as those with HIV/AIDS, solid organ transplantation, or hematological malignancies. CMV esophagitis typically presents with subacute or chronic symptoms, including odynophagia, dysphagia, weight loss, and fever. Endoscopic findings may include linear or serpiginous ulcers with raised borders and surrounding inflammation, and diagnosis is established by histopathological examination demonstrating characteristic cytoplasmic and nuclear inclusions consistent with CMV infection.

4. Fungal Infections (Non-Candida):

In addition to Candida species, other fungal pathogens such as Aspergillus species, Cryptococcus neoformans, Histoplasma capsulatum, and Pneumocystis jirovecii can cause infectious esophagitis, particularly in immunocompromised individuals with impaired cellular immunity or underlying pulmonary disease. Fungal esophagitis may present with nonspecific symptoms such as dysphagia, odynophagia, or retrosternal discomfort and may be associated with systemic fungal infections or disseminated disease. Diagnosis is established by endoscopic evaluation with biopsy and confirmed by histopathological examination, fungal culture, or molecular testing.

5. Bacterial Infections:

Bacterial esophagitis is relatively uncommon but can occur secondary to esophageal instrumentation, chemical injury, or underlying motility disorders that predispose to bacterial overgrowth. Common bacterial pathogens implicated in infectious esophagitis include Streptococcus species, Staphylococcus aureus, Escherichia coli, Klebsiella pneumoniae, and Mycobacterium tuberculosis. Bacterial esophagitis may present with symptoms such as odynophagia, dysphagia, fever, or chest pain and may be associated with underlying risk factors such as immunosuppression, esophageal strictures, or GERD.

Diagnosis is established by endoscopic evaluation with biopsy and confirmed by microbiological culture or histopathological examination of tissue specimens.

6. Parasitic Infections:

Parasitic esophagitis is rare but can occur in individuals with a history of travel to endemic regions or immunocompromised states. Parasitic pathogens implicated in esophagitis include Schistosoma species, Strongyloides stercoralis, Toxoplasma gondii, and Acanthamoeba species. Parasitic esophagitis may present with nonspecific symptoms such as dysphagia, odynophagia, or epigastric pain and may be associated with systemic parasitic infections or disseminated disease. Diagnosis is established by endoscopic evaluation with biopsy and confirmed by histopathological examination, serological testing, or molecular diagnostics.

Conclusion:

Common pathogens and opportunistic infections play a significant role in the etiology of infectious esophagitis, particularly in immunocompromised individuals or those with underlying predisposing factors. Candida species, herpes simplex virus (HSV), cytomegalovirus (CMV), and other fungal, bacterial, and parasitic pathogens can cause inflammation and mucosal injury in the esophagus, leading to a range of clinical manifestations and complications. Prompt recognition, accurate diagnosis, and targeted antimicrobial therapy are essential for managing infectious esophagitis and preventing complications such as strictures, perforation, or dissemination of infection. Multidisciplinary approaches involving gastroenterologists, infectious disease specialists, and immunologists are often required for comprehensive evaluation and management of infectious esophagitis.

Clinical Presentation and Diagnostic Approach

Infectious esophagitis presents a diverse array of clinical symptoms and requires a comprehensive diagnostic approach to accurately identify the underlying etiology. Understanding the clinical presentation and diagnostic strategies is essential for effective management and improved patient outcomes.

Clinical Presentation:

Infectious esophagitis manifests with various symptoms, often overlapping with other esophageal conditions, making diagnosis challenging. The clinical presentation typically includes:

1. **Dysphagia:** Difficulty swallowing is a common symptom, ranging from mild discomfort to severe pain upon swallowing. Patients may report food getting stuck in the throat or chest, leading to discomfort and impaired nutrition intake.
2. **Odynophagia:** Painful swallowing, known as odynophagia, is a hallmark symptom of esophagitis. Patients experience sharp, burning pain while swallowing, often localized to the chest or throat. This symptom is more indicative of mucosal inflammation and ulceration.
3. **Retrosternal Pain:** Patients may complain of retrosternal discomfort or pain behind the breastbone, resembling heartburn. This symptom can be confused with gastroesophageal reflux disease (GERD) or cardiac chest pain, highlighting the importance of a thorough

differential diagnosis.
4. **Systemic Symptoms:** In severe cases or immunocompromised individuals, infectious esophagitis may present with systemic symptoms such as fever, malaise, or weight loss. These manifestations indicate a more widespread infection or underlying immunodeficiency.

The clinical presentation of infectious esophagitis varies depending on the causative pathogen, underlying immune status, and presence of predisposing factors. Therefore, a detailed history and physical examination are crucial for identifying potential risk factors and guiding further diagnostic evaluation.

Diagnostic Approach:

Accurate diagnosis of infectious esophagitis requires a stepwise approach, integrating clinical assessment, endoscopic evaluation, and microbiological testing. The diagnostic algorithm typically involves the following steps:

1. **Clinical Evaluation:** A thorough history should focus on eliciting symptoms suggestive of esophageal pathology, such as dysphagia, odynophagia, or retrosternal pain. Clinicians should inquire about underlying medical conditions, immunosuppressive therapy, recent travel history, or high-risk behaviors that may predispose to infectious esophagitis.
2. **Endoscopic Evaluation:** Esophagogastroduodenoscopy (EGD) is the cornerstone of diagnostic evaluation for esophageal disorders, allowing direct visualization of the esophageal mucosa and collection of biopsy specimens. Endoscopic findings, including mucosal erythema, ulcerations, or exudates, provide valuable clues to the underlying etiology of esophagitis.

3. **Biopsy and Histopathology:** Tissue biopsy specimens obtained during endoscopy are essential for confirming the diagnosis of infectious esophagitis and identifying the causative pathogen. Histopathological examination of biopsy specimens enables the detection of characteristic morphological features such as fungal hyphae, viral inclusions, or bacterial colonies within the esophageal mucosa.
4. **Microbiological Testing:** Microbiological culture, polymerase chain reaction (PCR), or antigen detection assays may be employed to identify specific infectious pathogens in biopsy specimens or body fluids. Microbiological testing allows for rapid and accurate diagnosis of viral, bacterial, fungal, or parasitic etiologies of esophagitis, facilitating targeted antimicrobial therapy.
5. **Serological Testing:** Serological testing for specific antibodies or antigens may be useful in diagnosing certain viral infections associated with esophagitis, such as herpes simplex virus (HSV) or cytomegalovirus (CMV). Serological assays measure the presence and titers of specific antibodies or antigens in serum or body fluids, providing supportive evidence of systemic or disseminated infection.
6. **Radiological Imaging:** In selected cases, radiological imaging modalities such as barium swallow or computed tomography (CT) may be used to evaluate structural abnormalities, strictures, or complications associated with infectious esophagitis. Radiological imaging can provide complementary information to endoscopic findings and aid in treatment planning.

The diagnostic approach to infectious esophagitis requires careful consideration of clinical findings, endoscopic features, and microbiological results to establish an accurate diagnosis and guide appropriate treatment. Collaboration between gastroenterologists, infectious disease specialists, and pathologists is often necessary to optimize patient care and outcomes.

In summary, infectious esophagitis presents with a spectrum of clinical symptoms, necessitating a systematic diagnostic approach for accurate identification of the underlying etiology. Integration of clinical assessment, endoscopic evaluation, and microbiological testing is essential for effective management and improved prognosis in patients with infectious esophagitis. Early diagnosis and prompt initiation of targeted antimicrobial therapy are crucial for preventing complications and optimizing patient outcomes.

Treatment Strategies and Prognosis

Effective management of infectious esophagitis relies on targeted treatment strategies tailored to the specific causative pathogen, severity of infection, and patient-related factors. Additionally, understanding the prognosis associated with different infectious agents is crucial for optimizing patient outcomes and preventing complications.

Treatment Strategies:

1. **Antifungal Therapy:** For Candida esophagitis, antifungal agents such as fluconazole, itraconazole, or voriconazole are the mainstay of treatment. Oral fluconazole is often preferred for uncomplicated cases, while intravenous therapy may be necessary for severe or refractory infections. Duration of antifungal

therapy depends on the severity of infection and immune status of the patient, with prolonged courses recommended for immunocompromised individuals.

2. **Antiviral Therapy:** Herpes simplex virus (HSV) and cytomegalovirus (CMV) esophagitis require treatment with specific antiviral agents. Acyclovir or valacyclovir is used for HSV esophagitis, while ganciclovir or valganciclovir is preferred for CMV esophagitis. Intravenous therapy may be necessary for severe infections or immunocompromised patients. Duration of antiviral therapy varies based on clinical response and resolution of symptoms.

3. **Antibacterial Therapy:** Bacterial esophagitis is less common but may occur secondary to esophageal instrumentation, chemical injury, or underlying motility disorders. Treatment involves targeted antibiotic therapy based on microbiological culture and sensitivity results. Empirical coverage with broad-spectrum antibiotics may be initiated pending culture results, with adjustment based on susceptibility testing.

4. **Supportive Care:** Symptomatic relief is an integral part of treatment for infectious esophagitis and may include pain management, hydration, and nutritional support. Patients with severe dysphagia or odynophagia may benefit from liquid or soft diet modifications to facilitate swallowing and reduce discomfort. Adequate hydration is essential to prevent dehydration, particularly in patients with systemic symptoms or compromised oral intake.

5. **Immune Reconstitution:** In immunocompromised patients with infectious esophagitis, efforts should be made to optimize immune function through antiretroviral therapy (in HIV/AIDS), immunosuppression reduction (in transplant

recipients), or administration of immune-modulating agents (e.g., granulocyte-colony stimulating factor). Immune reconstitution therapy aims to enhance host defenses against opportunistic infections and improve treatment outcomes.

6. **Endoscopic Interventions:** In cases of severe esophageal strictures or complications such as hemorrhage or perforation, endoscopic interventions may be necessary to alleviate symptoms and prevent further morbidity. Endoscopic dilation, hemostasis, or stent placement may be performed under direct visualization to restore luminal patency and control bleeding.

Prognosis:

The prognosis of infectious esophagitis varies depending on several factors, including the underlying etiology, immune status of the patient, severity of infection, and timely initiation of appropriate treatment. Generally, the prognosis is favorable with prompt diagnosis and targeted antimicrobial therapy, leading to resolution of symptoms and mucosal healing. However, certain infectious agents may be associated with more severe or refractory disease courses, necessitating prolonged treatment and close monitoring for complications.

1. **Candida Esophagitis:** With appropriate antifungal therapy, Candida esophagitis typically responds well, especially in immunocompetent individuals. However, in immunocompromised patients or those with underlying risk factors, such as poorly controlled diabetes or prolonged corticosteroid use, recurrent or refractory infections may occur, requiring long-term maintenance therapy.

2. **Viral Esophagitis (HSV, CMV):** Herpes simplex virus (HSV) and cytomegalovirus (CMV) esophagitis may

have a more protracted course, particularly in immunocompromised patients. Early initiation of antiviral therapy is crucial to prevent dissemination of infection and improve outcomes. In severe cases, viral esophagitis may be associated with complications such as esophageal strictures, perforation, or systemic dissemination, which can impact prognosis and long-term morbidity.

3. **Bacterial Esophagitis:** Bacterial esophagitis is relatively uncommon and often responds well to targeted antibiotic therapy. However, severe infections or complications such as perforation or mediastinitis may occur, leading to increased morbidity and mortality. Timely diagnosis and appropriate antibiotic selection are essential for favorable treatment outcomes.

4. **Complications and Long-Term Sequelae:** Complications of infectious esophagitis, such as esophageal strictures, perforation, or systemic dissemination, can significantly impact prognosis and long-term quality of life. Close monitoring for complications and timely intervention are crucial for preventing adverse outcomes and optimizing patient recovery.

In conclusion, effective management of infectious esophagitis requires a multidisciplinary approach integrating targeted antimicrobial therapy, supportive care, and endoscopic interventions as needed. Prognosis varies depending on the underlying etiology and severity of infection, with early diagnosis and prompt initiation of appropriate treatment essential for improving outcomes and preventing complications. Long-term follow-up is necessary to monitor for recurrence, assess treatment response, and address any residual complications to ensure optimal patient care and quality of life.

CHAPTER 5: EOSINOPHILIC ESOPHAGITIS (EOE)

Definition and Clinical Features

Eosinophilic esophagitis (EoE) is a chronic immune-mediated inflammatory disorder of the esophagus characterized by eosinophilic infiltration of the esophageal mucosa. This condition was first described in the early 1990s and has since emerged as a significant cause of esophageal dysfunction, particularly in children and young adults. Understanding the definition, clinical features, and diagnostic criteria of EoE is crucial for accurate diagnosis and effective management of this condition.

Definition:

Eosinophilic esophagitis is defined as a chronic, immune-mediated inflammatory disorder of the esophagus characterized by the presence of eosinophils in the esophageal mucosa, typically in the absence of gastroesophageal reflux disease (GERD) or other causes of esophageal eosinophilia. The hallmark histological feature of EoE is the presence of ≥15 eosinophils per high-power field (HPF) on esophageal biopsy specimens obtained during upper endoscopy, despite proton pump inhibitor (PPI) therapy for at least 8 weeks to exclude PPI-responsive esophageal eosinophilia (PPI-REE).

Clinical Features:

Eosinophilic esophagitis presents with a spectrum of clinical features that vary depending on the age of onset, severity of inflammation, and duration of the disease. The clinical presentation may include:

1. **Dysphagia:** Dysphagia, or difficulty swallowing, is the most common symptom of EoE and often presents as intermittent episodes of food impaction or sticking in the esophagus. Patients may describe a sensation of food getting stuck in the chest or throat, particularly with solid foods, and may need to drink fluids or induce vomiting to relieve the obstruction.
2. **Food Impaction:** EoE is frequently associated with episodes of food impaction, particularly in children and adolescents. Food impaction occurs when ingested food becomes trapped in the esophagus due to narrowing or stricture formation secondary to chronic inflammation and fibrosis. Food impaction typically presents as acute chest pain, dysphagia, or choking, requiring urgent medical attention for endoscopic removal of the impacted food bolus.
3. **Reflux-like Symptoms:** Eosinophilic esophagitis may mimic symptoms of gastroesophageal reflux disease (GERD), including heartburn, regurgitation, or retrosternal discomfort. However, unlike GERD, EoE is typically unresponsive to acid suppression therapy with proton pump inhibitors (PPIs) and may require additional diagnostic evaluation to differentiate between the two conditions.

4. **Feeding Difficulties (Pediatric Patients):** In infants and young children, EoE may present with feeding difficulties, failure to thrive, or recurrent vomiting. These symptoms may be attributed to esophageal inflammation, strictures, or food aversion secondary to dysphagia or discomfort during feeding.

5. **Abdominal Pain:** Some patients with EoE may experience nonspecific abdominal pain or discomfort, particularly in children and adolescents. Abdominal pain may be related to esophageal dysmotility, visceral hypersensitivity, or secondary functional gastrointestinal disorders coexisting with EoE.

6. **Atopic Comorbidities:** Eosinophilic esophagitis is frequently associated with atopic conditions such as asthma, allergic rhinitis, atopic dermatitis, and food allergies, suggesting a shared immune-mediated pathogenesis. Patients with EoE may have a personal or family history of atopic disorders, highlighting the importance of comprehensive evaluation and management of concurrent allergic conditions.

7. **Extraesophageal Manifestations:** In addition to esophageal symptoms, EoE may manifest with extraesophageal symptoms such as chronic cough, throat clearing, or hoarseness, particularly in adults. These symptoms result from reflux of esophageal contents into the upper airway or larynx, leading to laryngopharyngeal reflux (LPR) and associated laryngeal inflammation.

The clinical features of EoE can vary widely among individuals and may overlap with other esophageal disorders, complicating the diagnostic process. A high index of suspicion is essential for recognizing EoE, particularly in patients with refractory esophageal symptoms, atopic comorbidities, or a family history of allergic disorders.

Diagnostic Approach:

The diagnosis of EoE requires a comprehensive evaluation integrating clinical assessment, endoscopic evaluation, and histological examination. The diagnostic algorithm typically includes the following steps:

1. **Clinical Assessment:** A thorough history and physical examination should focus on eliciting symptoms suggestive of esophageal dysfunction, including dysphagia, food impaction, or reflux-like symptoms. Attention should be paid to atopic comorbidities, family history of allergic disorders, and response to previous therapies.
2. **Endoscopic Evaluation:** Esophagogastroduodenoscopy (EGD) with biopsy is essential for assessing esophageal mucosal integrity and obtaining tissue specimens for histological examination. Endoscopic findings in EoE may include longitudinal furrows, concentric rings (trachealization), white plaques or exudates (pseudomembranes), esophageal strictures, or friability of the mucosa.
3. **Histological Examination:** Histological examination of esophageal biopsy specimens is necessary to confirm the diagnosis of EoE and assess the degree of eosinophilic inflammation. The presence of ≥15 eosinophils per high-power field (HPF) on esophageal biopsy specimens, despite PPI therapy for at least 8 weeks to exclude PPI-responsive esophageal eosinophilia (PPI-REE), supports the diagnosis of EoE.
4. **Additional Testing:** Additional diagnostic tests such as esophageal manometry, pH monitoring, or allergy testing may be performed to evaluate esophageal motility, assess acid reflux, or identify specific food

triggers contributing to EoE. These tests may provide valuable information for guiding treatment decisions and dietary modifications in patients with EoE.

In summary, eosinophilic esophagitis is a chronic immune-mediated inflammatory disorder of the esophagus characterized by eosinophilic infiltration of the esophageal mucosa. The clinical features of EoE are diverse and may include dysphagia, food impaction, reflux-like symptoms, feeding difficulties (in pediatric patients), atopic comorbidities, and extraesophageal manifestations. A comprehensive diagnostic approach integrating clinical assessment, endoscopic evaluation, and histological examination is essential for accurate diagnosis and effective management of EoE. Early recognition and intervention are crucial for improving patient outcomes and preventing complications associated with this chronic inflammatory condition.

Etiology and Immunopathogenesis

Eosinophilic esophagitis (EoE) is a complex immune-mediated disorder characterized by chronic inflammation of the esophagus, primarily driven by aberrant immune responses to dietary antigens and environmental triggers. Understanding the multifactorial etiology and immunopathogenesis of EoE is crucial for elucidating disease mechanisms, identifying potential therapeutic targets, and developing targeted treatment strategies.

Etiology:

The etiology of EoE is multifactorial, involving genetic predisposition, environmental factors, dysregulated immune responses, and interactions between the epithelium and mucosal immune system. Several key factors contribute to the pathogenesis of EoE:

1. **Genetic Susceptibility:** EoE has a strong genetic component, with evidence of familial aggregation and heritability. Genome-wide association studies (GWAS) have identified multiple susceptibility loci associated with EoE, including genes involved in epithelial barrier function (e.g., FLG, DSG1), immune regulation (e.g., CAPN14, CCL26), and allergic inflammation (e.g., TSLP, IL-13). These genetic variants may predispose individuals to epithelial dysfunction, impaired immune regulation, and heightened allergic responses, contributing to the development of EoE.

2. **Environmental Triggers:** Environmental factors play a critical role in triggering and exacerbating EoE, including dietary antigens, aeroallergens, microbial agents, and other environmental allergens. Common dietary triggers implicated in EoE include milk, wheat, soy, eggs, peanuts, and seafood, with elimination diets often used as a therapeutic approach to identify and avoid specific food allergens triggering disease flares. Aeroallergens such as pollen, dust mites, and animal dander may also exacerbate EoE symptoms in sensitized individuals, highlighting the importance of environmental allergen avoidance strategies.

3. **Epithelial Barrier Dysfunction:** Disruption of the esophageal epithelial barrier is a hallmark feature of EoE, leading to increased permeability, impaired mucosal integrity, and enhanced antigen exposure to the underlying immune cells. Epithelial barrier dysfunction may result from genetic mutations affecting structural proteins (e.g., filaggrin, desmoglein-1), dysregulated expression of

tight junction proteins (e.g., claudins, occludins), or exposure to environmental insults (e.g., allergens, acid reflux). Loss of barrier integrity allows allergens and inflammatory mediators to penetrate the mucosa, triggering immune activation and eosinophilic inflammation.

4. **Dysregulated Immune Responses:** EoE is characterized by dysregulated immune responses involving T-helper type 2 (Th2) cytokines, eosinophilic infiltration, mast cell activation, and IgE-mediated hypersensitivity reactions. Th2 cytokines such as interleukin-4 (IL-4), IL-5, and IL-13 play a central role in promoting allergic inflammation, eosinophil recruitment, and tissue remodeling in EoE. Eosinophils release pro-inflammatory mediators such as eosinophil cationic protein (ECP), major basic protein (MBP), and eosinophil-derived neurotoxin (EDN), contributing to tissue damage, fibrosis, and functional impairment of the esophagus.

5. **Microbial Dysbiosis:** Alterations in the esophageal microbiota, known as microbial dysbiosis, have been implicated in the pathogenesis of EoE, although the precise mechanisms remain unclear. Dysbiosis may result from disrupted epithelial barrier function, altered mucosal immunity, or environmental exposures to microbial antigens. Changes in the composition and diversity of the esophageal microbiota may influence immune homeostasis, exacerbate allergic inflammation, or modulate responses to dietary antigens, contributing to the development or progression of EoE.

Immunopathogenesis:

The immunopathogenesis of EoE involves a complex interplay between innate and adaptive immune responses, culminating in chronic eosinophilic inflammation and tissue remodeling within the esophagus. Key immunological processes implicated in EoE pathogenesis include:

1. **Antigen Sensitization:** Sensitization to dietary antigens and environmental allergens is a critical initiating event in EoE pathogenesis, leading to the activation of allergen-specific immune responses. Antigens are recognized by antigen-presenting cells (APCs) such as dendritic cells (DCs) or macrophages, which process and present antigenic peptides to naïve T cells in the context of major histocompatibility complex (MHC) molecules.
2. **T-Cell Activation:** Antigen presentation to naïve T cells results in T-cell activation and differentiation into effector T-cell subsets, including Th2 cells, Th17 cells, and regulatory T cells (Tregs). Th2 cells play a central role in promoting allergic inflammation in EoE by producing cytokines such as IL-4, IL-5, and IL-13, which stimulate B-cell activation, eosinophil recruitment, and immunoglobulin class switching to IgE.
3. **Eosinophilic Infiltration:** Th2 cytokines and chemokines orchestrate the recruitment and activation of eosinophils within the esophageal mucosa, leading to eosinophilic inflammation and tissue damage. Eosinophils release cytotoxic granule proteins, pro-inflammatory cytokines, and lipid mediators that amplify local inflammation, induce epithelial cell apoptosis, and contribute to tissue fibrosis and remodeling.
4. **Mast Cell Activation:** Mast cells are activated by allergen cross-linking of IgE antibodies bound to their surface, leading to degranulation and release of inflammatory mediators such as histamine,

leukotrienes, and prostaglandins. Mast cell-derived mediators contribute to vasodilation, smooth muscle contraction, mucus secretion, and recruitment of inflammatory cells, exacerbating tissue inflammation and hypersensitivity reactions in EoE.

5. **Epithelial Barrier Dysfunction:** Dysregulated immune responses and chronic inflammation disrupt the integrity of the esophageal epithelial barrier, leading to increased permeability, impaired mucosal repair, and enhanced antigen exposure to the underlying immune cells. Epithelial barrier dysfunction exacerbates allergen penetration, immune activation, and eosinophilic infiltration, perpetuating a cycle of inflammation and tissue damage in EoE.

6. **Fibrosis and Tissue Remodeling:** Prolonged inflammation and tissue injury in EoE can lead to esophageal fibrosis, subepithelial fibroblast proliferation, and extracellular matrix deposition, resulting in structural changes and functional alterations within the esophagus. Fibrosis and tissue remodeling may lead to esophageal strictures, narrowing of the esophageal lumen, and impaired esophageal motility, contributing to dysphagia, food impaction, and other symptoms of EoE.

In summary, eosinophilic esophagitis is a complex immune-mediated disorder characterized by chronic inflammation of the esophagus, driven by aberrant immune responses to dietary antigens and environmental triggers. The multifactorial etiology and immunopathogenesis of EoE involve genetic predisposition, environmental factors, epithelial barrier dysfunction, dysregulated immune responses, eosinophilic infiltration, mast cell activation, and tissue remodeling. Elucidating the underlying mechanisms of EoE pathogenesis is essential for developing targeted therapies aimed at modulating immune responses, restoring epithelial barrier function, and preventing disease progression in affected individuals.

Diagnostic Evaluation and Criteria

Accurate diagnosis of eosinophilic esophagitis (EoE) requires a comprehensive evaluation integrating clinical assessment, endoscopic findings, histological examination, and exclusion of other potential causes of esophageal eosinophilia. Understanding the diagnostic criteria and evaluation strategies is crucial for identifying individuals with EoE, initiating appropriate treatment, and monitoring disease progression.

Diagnostic Criteria:

The diagnosis of EoE is based on a combination of clinical symptoms, endoscopic findings, and histological evidence of eosinophilic inflammation in the esophageal mucosa. Key diagnostic criteria for EoE include:

1. **Clinical Symptoms:** Patients with EoE typically present with symptoms of esophageal dysfunction, such as dysphagia, food impaction, or reflux-like symptoms. Other common symptoms may include feeding difficulties (in pediatric patients), abdominal pain, and atopic comorbidities such as asthma or allergic rhinitis. Clinical symptoms may vary depending on the age of onset, severity of inflammation, and duration of the disease.
2. **Endoscopic Findings:** Esophagogastroduodenoscopy (EGD) with biopsy is essential for assessing esophageal mucosal integrity and identifying characteristic

endoscopic features of EoE. Endoscopic findings in EoE may include longitudinal furrows, concentric rings (trachealization), white plaques or exudates (pseudomembranes), esophageal strictures, or friability of the mucosa. These findings are suggestive of chronic inflammation and tissue remodeling within the esophagus.

3. **Histological Examination:** Histological evaluation of esophageal biopsy specimens is necessary to confirm the diagnosis of EoE and assess the degree of eosinophilic inflammation. The hallmark histological feature of EoE is the presence of ≥15 eosinophils per high-power field (HPF) on esophageal biopsy specimens obtained during upper endoscopy. Eosinophils are typically distributed throughout the esophageal mucosa, including the epithelium, lamina propria, and muscularis mucosae.

4. **Exclusion of Other Causes:** The diagnosis of EoE requires exclusion of other potential causes of esophageal eosinophilia, including gastroesophageal reflux disease (GERD), proton pump inhibitor-responsive esophageal eosinophilia (PPI-REE), eosinophilic gastroenteritis, and other eosinophilic gastrointestinal disorders. Additional diagnostic testing may be necessary to differentiate between EoE and other conditions presenting with similar clinical or histological features.

Diagnostic Evaluation:

The diagnostic evaluation of EoE typically involves the following steps:

1. **Clinical Assessment:** A detailed history and physical examination should focus on eliciting symptoms suggestive of esophageal dysfunction,

atopic comorbidities, dietary triggers, and response to previous therapies. Patient-reported symptoms such as dysphagia, food impaction, or reflux-like symptoms should be carefully documented to guide further diagnostic evaluation.

2. **Endoscopic Evaluation:** Esophagogastroduodenoscopy (EGD) with biopsy is the gold standard diagnostic modality for assessing esophageal mucosal integrity and identifying characteristic endoscopic features of EoE. Endoscopic findings such as longitudinal furrows, concentric rings, white plaques, or strictures provide valuable clues to the underlying pathology and guide targeted biopsy sampling for histological examination.

3. **Biopsy and Histopathology:** Tissue biopsy specimens obtained during EGD are essential for confirming the diagnosis of EoE and assessing the degree of eosinophilic inflammation. Multiple biopsy specimens should be obtained from the proximal and distal esophagus to ensure adequate sampling and minimize sampling variability. Histological examination of biopsy specimens allows for visualization of eosinophils, basal zone hyperplasia, papillary elongation, and other histological features characteristic of EoE.

4. **Microscopic Evaluation:** Histological examination of esophageal biopsy specimens should be performed by an experienced pathologist familiar with the histopathological criteria for EoE diagnosis. The presence of ≥ 15 eosinophils per high-power field (HPF) on esophageal biopsy specimens is a key diagnostic criterion for EoE. Additional histological features such as eosinophil microabscesses, basal zone hyperplasia, and subepithelial fibrosis may support the diagnosis of EoE but are not required for diagnosis.

5. **Exclusion of Other Causes:** Additional diagnostic testing may be necessary to exclude other potential causes of esophageal eosinophilia, particularly gastroesophageal reflux disease (GERD) and proton pump inhibitor-responsive esophageal eosinophilia (PPI-REE). Esophageal pH monitoring, impedance testing, or PPI trials may be performed to assess for evidence of acid reflux and response to acid suppression therapy. Other diagnostic tests such as allergy testing, stool studies, or imaging studies may be indicated based on clinical suspicion of alternative diagnoses.

Diagnostic Criteria and Scoring Systems:

Several diagnostic criteria and scoring systems have been proposed to standardize the diagnosis and assessment of EoE severity, including:

1. **The 2011 Updated Consensus Recommendations for Eosinophilic Esophagitis (EoE-UCR):** This consensus statement established diagnostic criteria for EoE, including clinical symptoms, endoscopic findings, and histological evidence of eosinophilic inflammation. According to the EoE-UCR, a diagnosis of EoE requires the presence of symptoms consistent with esophageal dysfunction, ≥15 eosinophils per high-power field (HPF) on esophageal biopsy, and exclusion of other causes of esophageal eosinophilia.
2. **The Eosinophilic Esophagitis Activity Index (EEsAI):** The EEsAI is a validated scoring system used to assess disease activity and severity in patients with EoE. The EEsAI incorporates clinical symptoms, endoscopic findings, histological features, and response to treatment to calculate a composite score reflecting disease activity and treatment response. The EEsAI

score ranges from 0 to 24, with higher scores indicating greater disease activity and severity.

3. **The Endoscopic Reference Score (EREFS):** The EREFS is an endoscopic scoring system used to assess endoscopic findings and severity in patients with EoE. The EREFS evaluates specific endoscopic features such as furrows, rings, exudates, and strictures, assigning a score based on the severity and extent of mucosal abnormalities observed during EGD. The EREFS score ranges from 0 to 9, with higher scores indicating greater endoscopic severity and mucosal involvement.

Conclusion:

Accurate diagnosis of eosinophilic esophagitis (EoE) requires a comprehensive evaluation integrating clinical assessment, endoscopic findings, histological examination, and exclusion of other potential causes of esophageal eosinophilia. Key diagnostic criteria for EoE include clinical symptoms consistent with esophageal dysfunction, endoscopic evidence of mucosal abnormalities, histological evidence of eosinophilic inflammation, and exclusion of other causes of esophageal eosinophilia. Standardized diagnostic criteria and scoring systems such as the EoE-UCR, EEsAI, and EREFS help to facilitate the diagnosis, assessment, and monitoring of disease activity and severity in patients with EoE. Early recognition and intervention are essential for improving patient outcomes and preventing complications associated with this chronic inflammatory condition.

Management Strategies: Pharmacological and Dietary

The management of eosinophilic esophagitis (EoE) involves a multifaceted approach aimed at reducing esophageal inflammation, alleviating symptoms, preventing complications, and improving quality of life. Pharmacological and dietary interventions play key roles in the management of EoE, targeting underlying inflammatory pathways, addressing food triggers, and optimizing nutritional status. A personalized treatment plan should be tailored to the individual patient based on disease severity, clinical symptoms, endoscopic findings, and response to therapy.

Pharmacological Management:

1. **Topical Corticosteroids:** Topical corticosteroids are the mainstay of pharmacological therapy for EoE and are effective in reducing esophageal inflammation and improving symptoms. Swallowed corticosteroids such as fluticasone propionate and budesonide are commonly used as first-line therapy for EoE, administered as an oral inhaler or viscous suspension. These medications are typically swallowed without inhalation to deliver the corticosteroid directly to the esophageal mucosa, minimizing systemic absorption and adverse effects.

2. **Proton Pump Inhibitors (PPIs):** Proton pump inhibitors (PPIs) may be used as adjunctive therapy in patients with EoE, particularly those with concomitant gastroesophageal reflux disease (GERD) or evidence of acid reflux on pH monitoring. PPIs help to reduce gastric acid secretion, alleviate reflux symptoms, and promote esophageal mucosal healing. In some cases, PPI therapy may improve esophageal eosinophilia and provide symptomatic relief, although the mechanism of action is not fully understood.

3. **Systemic Corticosteroids:** Systemic corticosteroids

such as prednisone or methylprednisolone may be considered for short-term management of severe or refractory EoE, particularly in patients with significant dysphagia, food impaction, or esophageal strictures. Systemic corticosteroids are effective in rapidly reducing esophageal inflammation and improving symptoms but are associated with potential systemic side effects and long-term complications, limiting their use as long-term maintenance therapy.

4. **Biologic Therapies:** Biologic therapies targeting specific inflammatory pathways have emerged as promising treatment options for EoE, particularly in patients with refractory disease or contraindications to corticosteroid therapy. Biologics such as anti-interleukin-5 (IL-5) monoclonal antibodies (e.g., mepolizumab, reslizumab) or anti-interleukin-13 (IL-13) monoclonal antibodies (e.g., dupilumab) target key cytokines involved in eosinophilic inflammation and tissue remodeling, offering targeted and personalized treatment approaches for EoE.

5. **Antifungal Therapy:** Antifungal agents such as fluconazole or itraconazole may be considered in patients with evidence of fungal colonization or refractory EoE, particularly those with concomitant fungal infections or oral thrush. Antifungal therapy aims to reduce fungal burden, suppress fungal overgrowth, and alleviate esophageal inflammation, although the role of antifungal therapy in EoE remains controversial and requires further investigation.

6. **Allergy Immunotherapy:** Allergy immunotherapy, including sublingual immunotherapy (SLIT) or subcutaneous immunotherapy (SCIT), may be considered in patients with evidence of allergic sensitization to specific food allergens or aeroallergens

contributing to EoE. Allergy immunotherapy aims to desensitize the immune system to allergen exposure, reduce allergic inflammation, and improve tolerance to specific allergens, offering potential long-term benefits in selected patients with EoE.

Dietary Management:

1. **Elimination Diets:** Elimination diets involve the systematic removal of specific food allergens from the diet based on allergy testing or empirical observation of symptom triggers. Common food allergens implicated in EoE include milk, wheat, soy, eggs, peanuts, tree nuts, fish, and shellfish. Elimination diets may be implemented as a first-line therapy or adjunctive therapy in patients with EoE, particularly those with evidence of food-triggered symptoms or allergic sensitization.
2. **Elemental Diet:** An elemental diet involves the exclusive consumption of nutritionally complete, hypoallergenic formulas containing predigested amino acids, carbohydrates, fats, vitamins, and minerals. Elemental diets provide complete nutritional support while eliminating potential food allergens and minimizing antigen exposure to the esophageal mucosa. Elemental diets are often used as a short-term induction therapy to achieve mucosal healing and symptom resolution in patients with severe or refractory EoE.
3. **Empiric Elimination Diets:** Empiric elimination diets involve the sequential removal of common food allergens from the diet without formal allergy testing, followed by gradual reintroduction and assessment of symptom response. Empiric elimination diets may be used in patients with suspected food-triggered symptoms or those who do not respond

to conventional therapies. Close monitoring and dietary supervision are essential to ensure nutritional adequacy and prevent unintended dietary restrictions or deficiencies.

4. **Targeted Elimination Diets:** Targeted elimination diets involve the identification and removal of specific food allergens based on allergy testing or dietary history, followed by strict avoidance to prevent symptom recurrence. Targeted elimination diets may be tailored to individual patient preferences, dietary restrictions, and cultural considerations, with the goal of minimizing allergen exposure and optimizing symptom control in patients with EoE.

5. **Nutritional Counseling:** Nutritional counseling and dietary education play a crucial role in the management of EoE, providing guidance on allergen avoidance, meal planning, label reading, and dietary modifications to optimize nutritional intake and minimize symptom triggers. Registered dietitians or nutritionists with expertise in EoE can work closely with patients to develop personalized dietary plans, identify hidden sources of allergens, and address nutritional deficiencies associated with dietary restrictions.

Integrated Approach:

The management of EoE often requires an integrated approach combining pharmacological therapy, dietary interventions, allergy testing, and multidisciplinary care to achieve optimal outcomes and improve quality of life for patients. Treatment strategies should be individualized based on disease severity, clinical symptoms, endoscopic findings, histological features, and response to therapy, with regular monitoring and follow-up to assess treatment efficacy, adjust therapy as needed, and prevent disease relapse or complications. Collaborative efforts among gastroenterologists, allergists, dietitians, and other healthcare providers are essential for coordinating care, addressing comorbidities, and optimizing long-term management of EoE.

In summary, the management of eosinophilic esophagitis (EoE) involves a comprehensive approach integrating pharmacological therapy, dietary interventions, allergy testing, and multidisciplinary care to reduce esophageal inflammation, alleviate symptoms, prevent complications, and improve quality of life. Pharmacological options include topical corticosteroids, proton pump inhibitors (PPIs), systemic corticosteroids, biologic therapies, antifungal therapy, and allergy immunotherapy, tailored to individual patient needs and treatment goals. Dietary interventions may include elimination diets, elemental diets, empiric elimination diets, targeted elimination diets, and nutritional counseling, aimed at identifying and avoiding food triggers, optimizing nutritional intake, and minimizing symptom recurrence. An integrated approach combining pharmacological and dietary interventions, along with regular monitoring and follow-up, is essential for achieving optimal outcomes and long-term management of EoE.

CHAPTER 6: CHEMICAL AND DRUG-INDUCED ESOPHAGITIS

Mechanisms of Injury

Esophagitis encompasses a spectrum of inflammatory conditions affecting the esophageal mucosa, characterized by varying degrees of mucosal injury, inflammation, and tissue damage. Understanding the mechanisms underlying esophageal injury is crucial for elucidating disease pathogenesis, identifying risk factors, and developing targeted therapeutic strategies. Several key mechanisms contribute to the pathophysiology of esophagitis, including gastroesophageal reflux, chemical injury, infectious agents, immune-mediated processes, and mechanical factors.

Gastroesophageal Reflux:

Gastroesophageal reflux disease (GERD) is one of the leading causes of esophagitis, characterized by the retrograde flow of gastric contents into the esophagus, leading to mucosal injury and inflammation. The mechanisms underlying GERD-related esophagitis include:

1. **Transient Relaxation of the Lower Esophageal Sphincter (LES):** The lower esophageal sphincter (LES) normally acts as a barrier preventing reflux of gastric contents into the esophagus. Transient relaxation of the LES, triggered by factors such as gastric distention, food intake, or hormonal fluctuations, allows for the reflux of acidic gastric contents into the esophagus, leading to mucosal injury.

2. **Decreased Lower Esophageal Sphincter Pressure:** Dysfunction of the LES, characterized by decreased pressure or impaired tone, predisposes individuals to GERD by impairing the integrity of the gastroesophageal barrier. Reduced LES pressure may result from factors such as obesity, hiatal hernia, medications, smoking, or dietary factors, increasing the risk of reflux and esophageal injury.

3. **Delayed Gastric Emptying:** Delayed gastric emptying, secondary to conditions such as gastroparesis or gastric outlet obstruction, prolongs the contact time between gastric contents and the esophageal mucosa, increasing the likelihood of acid reflux and mucosal injury. Delayed gastric emptying may exacerbate GERD symptoms and contribute to the development of esophagitis.

4. **Acid and Pepsin Exposure:** Acid and pepsin are major components of gastric contents that contribute to esophageal injury in GERD. Acidic refluxate, with a pH less than 4, causes direct chemical injury to the esophageal mucosa, leading to epithelial damage, inflammation, and ulceration. Pepsin, a proteolytic enzyme activated by acidic pH, further exacerbates mucosal injury by digesting proteins and disrupting

cellular integrity.
5. **Impaired Esophageal Clearance:** Impaired esophageal clearance, characterized by ineffective esophageal peristalsis or esophageal dysmotility, impairs the ability of the esophagus to clear refluxate, leading to prolonged mucosal exposure and increased risk of esophageal injury. Conditions such as esophageal dysmotility disorders, systemic sclerosis, or neuromuscular diseases may predispose individuals to impaired esophageal clearance and GERD-related complications.

Chemical Injury:

Chemical injury to the esophagus can result from exposure to caustic substances, corrosive agents, or irritants, leading to direct mucosal damage and inflammation. Common sources of chemical injury include:

1. **Acidic or Alkaline Ingestion:** Accidental or intentional ingestion of acidic or alkaline substances, such as household cleaners, industrial chemicals, or corrosive liquids, can cause severe esophageal injury and chemical burns. Acidic substances (pH < 2.5) cause coagulative necrosis and liquefactive necrosis, while alkaline substances (pH > 11.5) cause saponification and liquefactive necrosis, resulting in mucosal ulceration, perforation, and stricture formation.
2. **Medications:** Certain medications, such as nonsteroidal anti-inflammatory drugs (NSAIDs), bisphosphonates, potassium chloride tablets, or oral iron supplements, can cause esophageal injury and inflammation, particularly when taken without adequate hydration or in a supine position. These medications may induce direct mucosal damage, promote mucosal irritation, or impair esophageal

motility, increasing the risk of pill-induced esophagitis or drug-induced injury.
3. **Chemotherapy and Radiation Therapy:** Chemotherapy agents and radiation therapy used in the treatment of malignancies can cause mucosal injury and inflammation in the esophagus, leading to acute esophagitis or radiation-induced esophagitis. Chemotherapeutic agents such as anthracyclines, taxanes, or alkylating agents may induce mucosal damage through direct cytotoxic effects or immune-mediated mechanisms, while radiation therapy causes epithelial injury, vascular damage, and fibrosis in the irradiated tissues.
4. **Reflux of Gastric Contents:** Reflux of acidic gastric contents into the esophagus, as seen in GERD, can cause chemical injury to the esophageal mucosa, leading to erosive esophagitis or ulceration. Acidic refluxate, containing hydrochloric acid and pepsin, directly damages the esophageal epithelium, disrupts cellular integrity, and promotes inflammation, contributing to mucosal injury and tissue damage.

Infectious Agents:

Infectious esophagitis can result from colonization or invasion of the esophageal mucosa by pathogenic microorganisms, including viruses, bacteria, fungi, or parasites. Common infectious agents implicated in esophagitis include:

1. **Herpes Simplex Virus (HSV):** Herpes simplex virus (HSV) esophagitis is a common cause of infectious esophagitis, particularly in immunocompromised individuals, such as those with human immunodeficiency virus (HIV) infection or solid organ transplant recipients. HSV esophagitis presents with painful ulcers, vesicles, or plaques on the esophageal

mucosa, often extending longitudinally along the length of the esophagus.
2. **Candida Species:** Candida esophagitis, caused by Candida species such as Candida albicans, is the most common form of fungal esophagitis, particularly in immunocompromised patients, those with esophageal motility disorders, or individuals receiving broad-spectrum antibiotics or corticosteroids. Candida esophagitis presents with white plaques, pseudomembranes, or erosions on the esophageal mucosa, often associated with odynophagia or dysphagia.
3. **Cytomegalovirus (CMV):** Cytomegalovirus (CMV) esophagitis is a frequent complication of systemic immunosuppression, such as in patients with HIV infection, solid organ transplant recipients, or hematopoietic stem cell transplant recipients. CMV esophagitis manifests as linear or serpiginous ulcers, often located in the mid to distal esophagus, with surrounding erythema and inflammation.
4. **Varicella-Zoster Virus (VZV):** Varicella-zoster virus (VZV) esophagitis, caused by reactivation of latent VZV infection, typically occurs in immunocompromised individuals, such as those with HIV infection or hematologic malignancies. VZV esophagitis presents with linear or serpiginous ulcers, similar to those seen in HSV esophagitis, often associated with prodromal symptoms such as fever, malaise, or rash.
5. **Other Pathogens:** Other infectious agents implicated in esophagitis include bacteria (e.g., Mycobacterium tuberculosis, Actinomyces species), parasites (e.g., Cryptosporidium, Strongyloides), or opportunistic pathogens (e.g., Pneumocystis jirovecii, Aspergillus species), particularly in immunocompromised hosts or individuals with underlying systemic conditions.

Immune-Mediated Processes:

Immune-mediated esophagitis encompasses a diverse group of inflammatory disorders characterized by dysregulated immune responses to dietary antigens, environmental triggers, or self-antigens, leading to mucosal inflammation and tissue damage. Common immune-mediated processes involved in esophagitis include:

1. **Eosinophilic Esophagitis (EoE):** Eosinophilic esophagitis (EoE) is a chronic immune-mediated disorder characterized by eosinophilic infiltration of the esophageal mucosa, driven by aberrant Th2-mediated immune responses to dietary antigens or environmental allergens. EoE is associated with atopic comorbidities, such as asthma or allergic rhinitis, and presents with symptoms of esophageal dysfunction, including dysphagia, food impaction, or reflux-like symptoms.
2. **Autoimmune Esophagitis:** Autoimmune esophagitis is a rare form of esophagitis characterized by autoimmune-mediated inflammation of the esophageal mucosa, often associated with systemic autoimmune diseases such as systemic sclerosis, systemic lupus erythematosus, or autoimmune polyendocrine syndromes. Autoimmune esophagitis may present with symptoms of esophageal dysfunction, dysphagia, or odynophagia, and may be associated with autoantibodies targeting esophageal antigens.
3. **Graft-versus-Host Disease (GVHD):** Graft-versus-host disease (GVHD) is a common complication of allogeneic hematopoietic stem cell transplantation, characterized by donor T-cell-mediated immune responses targeting host tissues, including the

gastrointestinal tract. Esophageal GVHD presents with mucosal inflammation, ulceration, and stricturing, often associated with other manifestations of GVHD, such as skin rash, liver dysfunction, or intestinal graft-versus-host disease.

4. **Eosinophilic Gastrointestinal Disorders (EGIDs):** Eosinophilic gastrointestinal disorders (EGIDs) encompass a spectrum of inflammatory conditions involving eosinophilic infiltration of the gastrointestinal tract, including EoE, eosinophilic gastritis, eosinophilic gastroenteritis, and eosinophilic colitis. EGIDs are characterized by dysregulated immune responses, allergic inflammation, and tissue eosinophilia, with variable clinical presentations depending on the location and extent of eosinophilic involvement.

Mechanical Factors:

Mechanical factors such as trauma, foreign body ingestion, or iatrogenic injury can cause direct injury to the esophageal mucosa, leading to mucosal abrasions, lacerations, or perforations. Common mechanical factors contributing to esophageal injury include:

1. **Food Impaction:** Food impaction, resulting from the ingestion of large food boluses or poorly chewed food particles, can cause mechanical obstruction of the esophagus, leading to mucosal injury, inflammation, and ulceration. Food impaction is commonly seen in patients with underlying esophageal motility disorders, such as achalasia, diffuse esophageal spasm, or scleroderma, and presents with symptoms of dysphagia, odynophagia, or chest pain.

2. **Foreign Body Ingestion:** Ingestion of foreign bodies, such as bones, pills, coins, or esophageal prostheses,

can cause mechanical trauma to the esophageal mucosa, leading to mucosal injury, perforation, or obstruction. Foreign body ingestion may occur accidentally, particularly in children, or intentionally, in the setting of psychiatric disorders or eating disorders, and requires prompt evaluation and management to prevent complications.

3. **Iatrogenic Injury:** Iatrogenic injury to the esophagus can occur as a result of diagnostic or therapeutic procedures, such as upper endoscopy, esophageal dilation, or esophageal stent placement. Esophageal injury may result from mucosal tears, perforations, or thermal injury during procedural manipulation, leading to mucosal inflammation, ulceration, or stricture formation. Iatrogenic injury requires prompt recognition and appropriate management to minimize complications and optimize outcomes.

In summary, esophagitis encompasses a diverse array of inflammatory conditions involving the esophageal mucosa, characterized by varying degrees of mucosal injury, inflammation, and tissue damage. Mechanisms of injury in esophagitis include gastroesophageal reflux, chemical injury, infectious agents, immune-mediated processes, and mechanical factors, each contributing to the pathophysiology of esophageal inflammation and tissue injury. Understanding the underlying mechanisms of esophageal injury is essential for guiding diagnostic evaluation, identifying risk factors, and developing targeted therapeutic strategies to mitigate mucosal damage, alleviate symptoms, and prevent complications associated with esophagitis.

Common Culprits and Exogenous Agents

Esophagitis can be triggered by a variety of endogenous and exogenous factors, including dietary allergens, medications, environmental irritants, infectious agents, and chemical substances. Understanding the common culprits and exogenous agents associated with esophagitis is essential for identifying potential triggers, implementing preventive measures, and optimizing treatment strategies.

Dietary Allergens:

1. **Food Proteins:** Certain dietary proteins have been implicated as common triggers of eosinophilic esophagitis (EoE) and allergic esophagitis, leading to immune-mediated inflammation and mucosal injury. Common food allergens associated with EoE include milk, wheat, soy, eggs, peanuts, tree nuts, fish, and shellfish. These allergens can elicit hypersensitivity reactions in susceptible individuals, driving eosinophilic infiltration and inflammatory responses within the esophageal mucosa.
2. **Food Additives:** Food additives such as artificial colors, flavors, preservatives, and emulsifiers may exacerbate esophageal inflammation and mucosal injury in individuals with esophagitis, particularly those with sensitivities or intolerances to specific additives. Common additives implicated in esophagitis include monosodium glutamate (MSG), tartrazine (Yellow 5), sodium benzoate, and sulfites, which may trigger allergic reactions or exacerbate existing

inflammation in the esophagus.

3. **Acidic and Spicy Foods:** Acidic and spicy foods, such as citrus fruits, tomatoes, vinegar, onions, garlic, peppers, and caffeinated beverages, can exacerbate symptoms of reflux esophagitis or non-erosive reflux disease (NERD), leading to mucosal irritation, dyspepsia, or heartburn. These foods may increase gastric acid secretion, lower esophageal sphincter (LES) pressure, or prolong esophageal exposure to acidic refluxate, contributing to mucosal injury and inflammation in susceptible individuals.

Medications:

1. **Nonsteroidal Anti-Inflammatory Drugs (NSAIDs):** Nonsteroidal anti-inflammatory drugs (NSAIDs), including aspirin, ibuprofen, naproxen, and diclofenac, are known to cause esophageal injury and mucosal damage, particularly when taken in high doses or for prolonged periods. NSAIDs can induce direct chemical injury to the esophageal mucosa, impair mucosal defense mechanisms, and exacerbate underlying gastroesophageal reflux, leading to erosive esophagitis or pill-induced esophagitis.

2. **Bisphosphonates:** Bisphosphonate medications, used for the treatment of osteoporosis or bone metastases, are associated with esophageal irritation, inflammation, and ulceration, particularly when taken improperly or without adequate hydration. Bisphosphonates can cause direct mucosal injury, esophageal ulceration, or stricturing, leading to symptoms of dysphagia, odynophagia, or retrosternal discomfort.

3. **Potassium Chloride Tablets:** Potassium chloride tablets, commonly used as potassium supplements or electrolyte replacements, can cause esophageal injury

and mucosal irritation, particularly when taken in large or uncoated formulations. Potassium chloride tablets can induce local irritation, ulceration, or stricturing of the esophageal mucosa, leading to symptoms of dysphagia, odynophagia, or chest pain.

4. **Oral Iron Supplements:** Oral iron supplements, used for the treatment of iron deficiency anemia, are associated with esophageal irritation, mucosal injury, and pill-induced esophagitis, particularly when taken in large or poorly dissolved formulations. Oral iron supplements can cause direct chemical injury to the esophageal mucosa, leading to mucosal ulceration, inflammation, or stricturing, and may exacerbate underlying gastroesophageal reflux.

Environmental Irritants:

1. **Tobacco Smoke:** Tobacco smoke contains numerous toxic compounds, including nicotine, tar, and carcinogens, which can irritate the esophageal mucosa and exacerbate symptoms of esophagitis. Smoking has been linked to an increased risk of gastroesophageal reflux, erosive esophagitis, Barrett's esophagus, and esophageal adenocarcinoma, highlighting the detrimental effects of tobacco exposure on esophageal health.

2. **Alcohol Consumption:** Excessive alcohol consumption can irritate the esophageal mucosa, lower esophageal sphincter (LES) pressure, and promote gastroesophageal reflux, leading to mucosal injury, inflammation, and erosive esophagitis. Chronic alcohol abuse is associated with an increased risk of esophageal complications, including esophagitis, esophageal varices, esophageal cancer, and alcoholic liver disease, highlighting the importance of moderation and responsible alcohol consumption.

Infectious Agents:

1. **Viruses:** Viral infections, such as herpes simplex virus (HSV), cytomegalovirus (CMV), and varicella-zoster virus (VZV), can cause esophagitis in immunocompromised individuals or those with impaired cellular immunity. Viral esophagitis typically presents with painful ulceration, vesicles, or plaques on the esophageal mucosa, often accompanied by systemic symptoms such as fever, malaise, or rash.
2. **Fungi:** Fungal infections, particularly candida species such as Candida albicans, can cause esophagitis in immunocompromised patients or those with underlying risk factors such as esophageal motility disorders or broad-spectrum antibiotic use. Candida esophagitis presents with white plaques, pseudomembranes, or erosions on the esophageal mucosa, often associated with symptoms of odynophagia, dysphagia, or retrosternal discomfort.
3. **Bacteria:** Bacterial infections, such as Mycobacterium tuberculosis, Actinomyces species, or Helicobacter pylori, can rarely cause esophagitis in immunocompromised hosts or individuals with underlying risk factors such as immunodeficiency, malnutrition, or systemic illnesses. Bacterial esophagitis typically presents with localized inflammation, ulceration, or abscess formation in the esophageal mucosa, often associated with systemic symptoms or predisposing conditions.

Chemical Substances:

1. **Caustic Substances:** Ingestion of caustic substances, such as household cleaners, industrial chemicals, or corrosive liquids, can cause severe esophageal injury,

chemical burns, and mucosal necrosis, leading to acute corrosive esophagitis or chemical esophageal strictures. Caustic esophageal injury requires immediate medical evaluation and management to minimize tissue damage and prevent complications such as perforation or stricture formation.

2. **Acidic or Alkaline Solutions:** Accidental or intentional ingestion of acidic or alkaline solutions, such as hydrochloric acid, sulfuric acid, or sodium hydroxide, can cause rapid and extensive esophageal injury, leading to chemical burns, tissue necrosis, and perforation. Acidic solutions cause coagulative necrosis, while alkaline solutions cause liquefactive necrosis, resulting in severe mucosal damage and potential life-threatening complications.

3. **Medicinal Formulations:** Certain medicinal formulations, such as concentrated syrups, effervescent tablets, or enteric-coated pills, may increase the risk of esophageal injury or pill-induced esophagitis due to delayed dissolution, prolonged esophageal contact time, or localized mucosal irritation. Patients should be advised to take medications with adequate hydration, in an upright position, and with food if indicated, to minimize the risk of esophageal injury or mucosal irritation.

In summary, esophagitis can be triggered by a variety of endogenous and exogenous factors, including dietary allergens, medications, environmental irritants, infectious agents, and chemical substances. Common culprits and exogenous agents associated with esophagitis include food allergens, NSAIDs, bisphosphonates, tobacco smoke, alcohol consumption, viral infections, fungal infections, bacterial infections, caustic substances, acidic or alkaline solutions, and medicinal formulations. Identifying and avoiding potential triggers, implementing preventive measures, and optimizing treatment strategies are essential for managing esophagitis and minimizing mucosal injury, inflammation, and complications associated with this inflammatory condition.

Clinical Presentation and Diagnostic Considerations

Esophagitis manifests with a diverse range of clinical presentations, varying from asymptomatic mucosal inflammation to severe complications such as esophageal strictures or perforation. Recognizing the clinical features and implementing appropriate diagnostic evaluations are crucial for accurately diagnosing esophagitis, identifying underlying etiologies, and guiding optimal management strategies.

Clinical Presentation:

1. **Dysphagia:** Dysphagia, or difficulty swallowing, is a common symptom of esophagitis, particularly in cases of severe mucosal inflammation, ulceration, or stricture formation. Patients may describe a sensation of food sticking in the chest or throat, discomfort or pain with swallowing, or the need to swallow repeatedly to clear food from the esophagus.
2. **Odynophagia:** Odynophagia, or painful swallowing, is another hallmark symptom of esophagitis, often associated with mucosal inflammation, ulceration, or erosions. Patients may experience sharp, burning, or stabbing pain with swallowing, localized to the chest or retrosternal area, which may worsen with ingestion of acidic or spicy foods.
3. **Retrosternal Discomfort:** Retrosternal discomfort, also known as retrosternal pain or chest pain, is

a common complaint in patients with esophagitis, particularly in cases of gastroesophageal reflux disease (GERD) or erosive esophagitis. Patients may describe a burning sensation or pressure-like discomfort in the retrosternal area, often exacerbated by lying down, bending over, or consuming acidic or fatty foods.

4. **Heartburn:** Heartburn, or pyrosis, is a classic symptom of GERD and reflux esophagitis, characterized by a burning sensation or discomfort in the chest or epigastric region, typically occurring after meals or when lying down. Heartburn may be accompanied by regurgitation of gastric contents, sour taste in the mouth, or belching, and is often relieved by antacids or proton pump inhibitors (PPIs).

5. **Regurgitation:** Regurgitation, or the reflux of gastric contents into the esophagus, is a common manifestation of GERD and reflux esophagitis, resulting in the sensation of fluid or food moving upward from the stomach into the throat or mouth. Patients may experience sour or bitter-tasting regurgitation, particularly when reclining or bending over, which may be associated with coughing or throat clearing.

6. **Dyspepsia:** Dyspepsia, or indigestion, is a nonspecific symptom often reported by patients with esophagitis, reflecting impaired digestion or discomfort in the upper gastrointestinal tract. Dyspeptic symptoms may include bloating, fullness, early satiety, epigastric pain, or nausea, which may overlap with symptoms of esophageal or gastric disorders.

7. **Alarm Symptoms:** Alarm symptoms such as unintentional weight loss, gastrointestinal bleeding, persistent vomiting, dysphagia to solids, or iron deficiency anemia may indicate underlying complications of esophagitis, such as esophageal

strictures, Barrett's esophagus, or esophageal adenocarcinoma, and require prompt evaluation and management.

Diagnostic Considerations:

1. **Upper Endoscopy:** Upper endoscopy, or esophagogastroduodenoscopy (EGD), is the gold standard diagnostic test for evaluating esophagitis, allowing direct visualization of the esophageal mucosa, identification of mucosal abnormalities, and acquisition of biopsy specimens for histological evaluation. Endoscopic findings suggestive of esophagitis include mucosal erythema, edema, erosions, ulcerations, or strictures, which may vary in severity depending on the underlying etiology.

2. **Histological Evaluation:** Histological examination of esophageal biopsy specimens obtained during upper endoscopy is essential for confirming the diagnosis of esophagitis, assessing the degree of mucosal inflammation, and identifying specific histopathological features associated with different etiologies. Histological findings consistent with esophagitis include increased eosinophilic infiltration, neutrophilic inflammation, basal cell hyperplasia, or epithelial changes such as elongation of papillae or loss of intercellular bridges.

3. **Esophageal pH Monitoring:** Esophageal pH monitoring is indicated in patients with suspected GERD or reflux esophagitis, particularly those with atypical symptoms, refractory disease, or inconclusive endoscopic findings. Ambulatory pH monitoring allows continuous measurement of esophageal pH over 24 to 48 hours, assessing the frequency, duration, and severity of acid reflux episodes, and correlating symptoms with acid exposure.

4. **Esophageal Manometry:** Esophageal manometry is useful for evaluating esophageal motility disorders, esophageal dysmotility, or impaired esophageal clearance in patients with esophagitis, particularly those with dysphagia, chest pain, or suspected esophageal motility disorders. Manometric studies assess esophageal peristalsis, lower esophageal sphincter (LES) function, and esophageal transit, providing valuable information on esophageal motor function and coordination.
5. **Barium Swallow:** Barium swallow, or esophagography, may be performed to assess esophageal anatomy, mucosal contour, luminal narrowing, or motility disorders in patients with suspected esophagitis, particularly when endoscopy is contraindicated or unavailable. Barium studies may reveal mucosal irregularities, strictures, ulcers, or filling defects suggestive of esophageal pathology.
6. **Laboratory Investigations:** Laboratory investigations such as complete blood count (CBC), liver function tests (LFTs), renal function tests (RFTs), and serological testing for infectious agents (e.g., herpes simplex virus, cytomegalovirus, candida) may be indicated in patients with suspected infectious esophagitis, immunocompromised individuals, or those with systemic symptoms suggestive of underlying pathology.
7. **Allergy Testing:** Allergy testing, including skin prick testing, serum IgE testing, or patch testing, may be considered in patients with suspected allergic esophagitis or eosinophilic esophagitis (EoE), particularly those with atopic comorbidities, allergic symptoms, or refractory disease. Allergy testing aims to identify potential triggers, such as food allergens or environmental allergens, that may contribute to

esophageal inflammation and mucosal injury.

In summary, esophagitis presents with a spectrum of clinical symptoms, ranging from dysphagia and odynophagia to retrosternal discomfort, heartburn, and regurgitation. Diagnostic evaluation of esophagitis involves a multidisciplinary approach, including upper endoscopy, histological examination, esophageal pH monitoring, manometric studies, barium swallow, and laboratory investigations, tailored to individual patient characteristics, symptomatology, and underlying etiologies. Early recognition, accurate diagnosis, and targeted management strategies are essential for optimizing outcomes and preventing complications associated with esophagitis.

Prevention and Management Approaches

Preventing esophagitis and effectively managing its symptoms and complications require a multifaceted approach addressing underlying causes, reducing risk factors, and implementing appropriate therapeutic interventions. Management strategies aim to alleviate symptoms, promote mucosal healing, prevent complications, and improve overall quality of life for patients with esophagitis.

Prevention Strategies:

1. **Dietary Modification:** Dietary modification plays a crucial role in preventing esophagitis, particularly in individuals with gastroesophageal reflux disease (GERD) or eosinophilic esophagitis (EoE). Patients should be advised to avoid trigger foods such as spicy, acidic, fatty, or allergenic foods that may exacerbate symptoms of reflux or allergic

inflammation. Maintaining a balanced diet with adequate fiber, hydration, and nutrient intake can help optimize gastrointestinal health and reduce the risk of esophageal irritation.
2. **Lifestyle Modifications:** Lifestyle modifications are essential for preventing esophagitis and minimizing symptoms of gastroesophageal reflux. Patients should be counseled to avoid smoking, limit alcohol consumption, maintain a healthy weight, and practice proper posture and sleeping habits to reduce intra-abdominal pressure and minimize reflux episodes. Elevating the head of the bed, avoiding late-night meals, and allowing sufficient time between meals and bedtime can help reduce nocturnal reflux and improve symptom control.
3. **Medication Management:** Medication management plays a central role in preventing esophagitis, particularly in patients with GERD or underlying medical conditions requiring long-term pharmacotherapy. Patients should be instructed to take medications as prescribed, adhere to recommended dosages and administration instructions, and avoid medications known to exacerbate esophageal irritation or mucosal injury, such as nonsteroidal anti-inflammatory drugs (NSAIDs) or potassium chloride tablets. Proton pump inhibitors (PPIs), histamine-2 receptor antagonists (H2RAs), and mucosal protectants may be prescribed to reduce gastric acid secretion, promote mucosal healing, and alleviate symptoms of reflux or erosive esophagitis.
4. **Weight Management:** Weight management is crucial for preventing esophagitis, particularly in individuals with obesity or abdominal adiposity, which can increase intra-abdominal pressure and predispose

to gastroesophageal reflux. Patients should be encouraged to achieve and maintain a healthy weight through a combination of dietary modifications, regular physical activity, and lifestyle changes aimed at reducing excess adiposity and improving metabolic health.

5. **Avoidance of Irritants:** Avoidance of irritants and potential triggers is essential for preventing esophagitis and minimizing mucosal injury. Patients should be educated about the harmful effects of tobacco smoke, environmental pollutants, chemical substances, and occupational hazards on esophageal health, and encouraged to avoid exposure to these irritants whenever possible. Occupational safety measures, environmental controls, and personal protective equipment may be recommended to minimize occupational or environmental exposures associated with esophageal irritation or mucosal injury.

Management Approaches:

1. **Pharmacological Therapy:** Pharmacological therapy plays a central role in managing esophagitis, with the primary goals of symptom relief, mucosal healing, and prevention of complications. Proton pump inhibitors (PPIs) are first-line agents for the treatment of GERD-related esophagitis, providing potent acid suppression, mucosal protection, and symptom relief. H2 receptor antagonists (H2RAs), antacids, alginate-based formulations, and mucosal protectants may be used as adjunctive therapies to provide additional symptom relief and promote mucosal healing in patients with mild to moderate esophagitis.

2. **Topical Steroids:** Topical steroids such as swallowed fluticasone or budesonide are recommended as first-

line therapy for eosinophilic esophagitis (EoE), aimed at reducing esophageal inflammation, eosinophilic infiltration, and mucosal fibrosis. Topical steroids are effective in inducing clinical and histological remission, improving dysphagia, and preventing disease recurrence in patients with EoE, particularly when combined with dietary elimination therapy or proton pump inhibitors (PPIs).

3. **Dietary Elimination Therapy:** Dietary elimination therapy plays a key role in managing EoE and allergic esophagitis, aimed at identifying and avoiding trigger foods that may exacerbate esophageal inflammation or allergic responses. Patients may undergo allergy testing or food elimination diets to identify potential allergens or sensitivities, followed by strict avoidance of trigger foods and adherence to hypoallergenic or elemental diets to minimize mucosal irritation and promote disease remission.

4. **Esophageal Dilation:** Esophageal dilation is indicated for the management of esophageal strictures or narrowing secondary to chronic inflammation, fibrosis, or scarring in patients with esophagitis. Endoscopic or bougie dilation procedures are performed to mechanically expand the narrowed esophageal lumen, improve dysphagia, and restore esophageal patency, allowing for improved swallowing function and symptom relief.

5. **Surgical Intervention:** Surgical intervention may be considered in select cases of refractory esophagitis, complications such as esophageal perforation or hemorrhage, or underlying structural abnormalities requiring corrective procedures. Antireflux surgery (e.g., fundoplication) may be performed to restore gastroesophageal competence, prevent reflux, and reduce the risk of recurrent esophagitis in patients

with GERD-related complications.

6. **Endoscopic Therapy:** Endoscopic therapy, including techniques such as endoscopic mucosal resection (EMR), endoscopic submucosal dissection (ESD), or endoscopic mucosal ablation, may be utilized for the management of early-stage esophageal neoplasms, dysplastic lesions, or Barrett's esophagus with high-grade dysplasia. Endoscopic therapy aims to achieve complete resection of neoplastic lesions, eradicate dysplastic epithelium, and prevent progression to invasive malignancy, offering a minimally invasive alternative to surgical resection.

7. **Follow-Up and Surveillance:** Follow-up and surveillance are essential components of esophagitis management, aimed at monitoring disease progression, assessing treatment response, and detecting complications such as strictures, Barrett's esophagus, or esophageal adenocarcinoma. Patients should undergo regular clinical evaluations, endoscopic surveillance, histological assessments, and imaging studies as indicated based on disease severity, underlying risk factors, and treatment modalities employed.

In summary, preventing esophagitis and effectively managing its symptoms and complications require a comprehensive approach addressing underlying causes, reducing risk factors, and implementing appropriate therapeutic interventions. Prevention strategies focus on dietary modification, lifestyle changes, weight management, avoidance of irritants, and medication management to minimize mucosal injury and promote esophageal health. Management approaches include pharmacological therapy, topical steroids, dietary elimination therapy, esophageal dilation, surgical intervention, endoscopic therapy, and follow-up surveillance, tailored to individual patient characteristics, disease severity, and underlying etiologies. Collaborative efforts between patients, healthcare providers, and multidisciplinary teams are essential for optimizing outcomes and improving quality of life for individuals with esophagitis.

CHAPTER 7: RADIATION ESOPHAGITIS

Pathophysiology and Radiation Injury

Esophagitis can result from various insults to the esophageal mucosa, including chemical, infectious, immune-mediated, mechanical, and radiation-induced injuries. Radiation injury to the esophagus, known as radiation esophagitis, occurs as a consequence of therapeutic radiation exposure to the chest or upper abdomen for the treatment of thoracic malignancies, mediastinal tumors, or metastatic disease. Understanding the pathophysiology of radiation-induced esophagitis is essential for optimizing prevention strategies, early detection, and management approaches in patients undergoing radiation therapy.

Pathophysiology of Radiation Esophagitis:

1. **Direct Cellular Damage:** Radiation therapy delivers ionizing radiation to target tissues, causing direct cellular damage to the esophageal epithelium,

submucosa, and muscular layers. Radiation-induced DNA damage, oxidative stress, and inflammatory responses lead to cell death, tissue injury, and disruption of mucosal integrity, predisposing to mucositis, ulceration, and inflammation in the irradiated esophagus.

2. **Endothelial Injury:** Radiation exposure induces endothelial injury and dysfunction in the esophageal microvasculature, disrupting capillary integrity, impairing tissue perfusion, and promoting microvascular thrombosis and ischemia. Endothelial cell damage leads to vascular congestion, edema, and submucosal hemorrhage, exacerbating tissue hypoxia, inflammation, and mucosal injury in the irradiated esophagus.

3. **Inflammatory Responses:** Radiation therapy triggers acute and chronic inflammatory responses in the irradiated esophagus, characterized by infiltration of inflammatory cells, release of proinflammatory cytokines, and activation of immune-mediated pathways. Inflammatory cell recruitment, including neutrophils, lymphocytes, and macrophages, contributes to tissue inflammation, immune activation, and tissue remodeling, further exacerbating mucosal injury and fibrosis in the irradiated esophagus.

4. **Fibrotic Remodeling:** Chronic radiation exposure induces fibrotic remodeling of the esophageal wall, characterized by excessive collagen deposition, myofibroblast activation, and tissue fibrosis. Fibrotic changes lead to progressive stiffening of the esophageal wall, narrowing of the esophageal lumen, and impaired esophageal motility, predisposing to dysphagia, stricture formation, and functional impairment in patients with radiation esophagitis.

5. **Impaired Mucosal Healing:** Radiation therapy impairs mucosal healing and regeneration in the irradiated esophagus, inhibiting epithelial cell proliferation, migration, and differentiation. Impaired mucosal turnover, delayed wound healing, and compromised barrier function prolong mucosal injury, exacerbate inflammation, and increase susceptibility to secondary infections, leading to prolonged symptoms and delayed recovery in patients with radiation-induced esophagitis.

Clinical Presentation of Radiation Esophagitis:

1. **Acute Phase:** Acute radiation esophagitis typically occurs within weeks to months following initiation of radiation therapy, presenting with symptoms of mucositis, dysphagia, odynophagia, chest pain, or retrosternal discomfort. Patients may experience acute inflammatory reactions, such as erythema, edema, and ulceration of the esophageal mucosa, often associated with systemic symptoms such as fatigue, anorexia, or weight loss.
2. **Chronic Phase:** Chronic radiation esophagitis may develop months to years after completion of radiation therapy, characterized by persistent or recurrent symptoms of dysphagia, chest pain, or food impaction. Chronic fibrotic changes, strictures, or stenosis of the esophagus may occur as late complications of radiation injury, leading to progressive functional impairment, swallowing difficulties, or obstructive symptoms in affected patients.

Diagnostic Considerations:

1. **Endoscopic Evaluation:** Endoscopic evaluation with esophagogastroduodenoscopy (EGD) is the

primary diagnostic modality for assessing radiation esophagitis, allowing direct visualization of the esophageal mucosa, identification of mucosal changes, and characterization of mucosal injury severity. Endoscopic findings may include erythema, edema, ulceration, friability, or strictures of the irradiated esophagus, correlating with the degree of radiation-induced mucosal damage.

2. **Histological Examination:** Histological examination of esophageal biopsy specimens obtained during endoscopy is essential for confirming the diagnosis of radiation esophagitis, assessing the degree of mucosal inflammation, and ruling out other etiologies of esophageal injury. Histological findings may include acute inflammatory changes, epithelial injury, submucosal fibrosis, or vascular damage consistent with radiation-induced mucosal injury.

3. **Radiological Imaging:** Radiological imaging studies such as barium swallow, computed tomography (CT) scan, or magnetic resonance imaging (MRI) may be performed to assess the extent of esophageal injury, evaluate for structural abnormalities, or detect complications such as strictures, fistulas, or perforation in patients with radiation esophagitis. Radiological findings may include esophageal wall thickening, luminal narrowing, or focal strictures indicative of radiation-induced mucosal injury.

Management Approaches:

1. **Symptomatic Relief:** Symptomatic relief of acute radiation esophagitis may be achieved with supportive measures such as pain management, hydration, nutritional support, and mucosal protection. Patients may benefit from topical anesthetics, viscous lidocaine, or oral analgesics to alleviate pain and

discomfort associated with mucositis or ulceration in the irradiated esophagus.

2. **Dietary Modifications:** Dietary modifications, including soft or liquid diet, avoidance of spicy or acidic foods, and frequent small meals, may help alleviate symptoms of dysphagia, odynophagia, or retrosternal discomfort in patients with radiation esophagitis. Nutritional supplementation, enteral feeding, or parenteral nutrition may be indicated for patients with severe dysphagia, weight loss, or malnutrition secondary to esophageal obstruction or functional impairment.

3. **Pharmacological Therapy:** Pharmacological therapy with proton pump inhibitors (PPIs), histamine-2 receptor antagonists (H2RAs), sucralfate, or prostaglandin analogs may be prescribed to reduce gastric acid secretion, promote mucosal healing, and alleviate symptoms of reflux or erosive esophagitis in patients with radiation-induced esophagitis. Topical corticosteroids or oral corticosteroid therapy may be considered for patients with severe inflammation, refractory symptoms, or progressive fibrotic changes in the irradiated esophagus.

4. **Endoscopic Interventions:** Endoscopic interventions such as esophageal dilation, stent placement, or endoscopic mucosal resection (EMR) may be performed to alleviate dysphagia, relieve luminal obstruction, or manage complications such as strictures or fistulas in patients with radiation esophagitis. Endoscopic therapy aims to improve esophageal patency, restore swallowing function, and optimize nutritional intake in affected individuals.

5. **Surgical Intervention:** Surgical intervention may be considered in select cases of refractory radiation esophagitis, complicated strictures, or persistent

symptoms requiring definitive management. Surgical options may include esophageal bypass procedures, esophagectomy, or reconstruction of the esophagus to alleviate dysphagia, improve quality of life, and prevent further complications in patients with advanced or unresectable disease.

In summary, radiation esophagitis is a common complication of therapeutic radiation exposure to the chest or upper abdomen, characterized by mucosal injury, inflammation, and fibrotic changes in the irradiated esophagus. Understanding the pathophysiology, clinical presentation, diagnostic considerations, and management approaches of radiation-induced esophagitis is essential for optimizing patient care, minimizing symptoms, and preventing complications associated with this radiation-related complication. Collaborative efforts between radiation oncologists, gastroenterologists, surgeons, and supportive care teams are essential for implementing preventive strategies, early detection, and targeted interventions to improve outcomes and quality of life for patients undergoing radiation therapy.

Clinical Presentation and Timing of Symptoms

The clinical presentation of esophagitis varies depending on the underlying etiology, severity of mucosal injury, and patient-specific factors. Understanding the timing of symptoms is crucial for identifying potential triggers, guiding diagnostic evaluations, and implementing appropriate management strategies in patients with esophagitis of various origins.

Clinical Presentation:

1. Acute Esophagitis:

Dysphagia: Dysphagia, or difficulty swallowing, is a hallmark symptom of acute esophagitis, characterized by a sensation of food sticking in the chest or throat, discomfort or pain with swallowing, or the need to swallow repeatedly to clear food from the esophagus. Dysphagia may be attributed to mucosal inflammation, edema, or ulceration, impairing esophageal transit and bolus clearance.

Odynophagia: Odynophagia, or painful swallowing, is a common complaint in acute esophagitis, reflecting mucosal irritation, ulceration, or erosions in the esophagus. Patients may experience sharp, burning, or stabbing pain with swallowing, localized to the chest or retrosternal area, which may worsen with ingestion of acidic or spicy foods.

Retrosternal Discomfort: Retrosternal discomfort, also known as retrosternal pain or chest pain, is frequently reported in acute esophagitis, particularly in cases of reflux esophagitis or infectious esophagitis. Patients may describe a burning sensation or pressure-like discomfort in the retrosternal area, exacerbated by lying down, bending over, or consuming acidic or fatty foods.

Heartburn and Regurgitation: Heartburn, or pyrosis, and regurgitation of gastric contents into the esophagus are classic symptoms of gastroesophageal reflux disease (GERD) and reflux esophagitis, commonly occurring after meals or when lying down. Heartburn may be accompanied by regurgitation of sour or bitter-tasting gastric contents, belching, or throat clearing, reflecting reflux of acid or bile into the esophagus.

Dyspepsia: Dyspeptic symptoms such as bloating, fullness, early satiety, epigastric pain, or nausea may be present in acute esophagitis, reflecting impaired digestion, gastric reflux, or mucosal irritation in the upper gastrointestinal tract. Dyspeptic symptoms may overlap with symptoms of esophageal or gastric disorders, warranting further evaluation and differential diagnosis.

2. **Chronic Esophagitis:**

Persistent Dysphagia: Chronic esophagitis may present with persistent or recurrent dysphagia, reflecting ongoing mucosal inflammation, fibrosis, or strictures in the esophagus. Patients may experience progressive narrowing of the esophageal lumen, impaired bolus transit, or obstructive symptoms requiring intervention to alleviate dysphagia and improve swallowing function.

Chronic Chest Pain: Chronic chest pain or retrosternal discomfort may persist in patients with chronic esophagitis, reflecting ongoing mucosal irritation, reflux episodes, or visceral hypersensitivity in the esophagus. Chronic chest pain may be exacerbated by certain foods, beverages, or activities and may be associated with anxiety, depression, or somatization disorders.

Recurrent Heartburn and Regurgitation: Recurrent episodes of heartburn, regurgitation, or belching may occur in patients with chronic esophagitis, particularly in cases of GERD or reflux-related complications. Persistent reflux symptoms may lead to erosive changes, Barrett's esophagus, or esophageal adenocarcinoma, necessitating long-term management and surveillance to prevent disease progression.

Weight Loss and Malnutrition: Weight loss, malnutrition, or nutritional deficiencies may develop in patients with severe or refractory esophagitis, resulting from dysphagia, odynophagia, anorexia, or impaired nutrient absorption. Chronic inflammation, mucosal injury, or strictures in the esophagus may compromise nutritional intake, necessitating dietary modification, enteral feeding, or nutritional supplementation to maintain adequate caloric intake and prevent complications of malnutrition.

Timing of Symptoms:

1. **Immediate Symptoms:** Some symptoms of esophagitis may occur immediately following exposure to triggering factors, such as ingestion of allergenic foods, acidic beverages, or caustic substances. Immediate symptoms may include acute dysphagia, odynophagia, retrosternal discomfort, or heartburn, reflecting direct mucosal injury, chemical irritation, or inflammatory responses in the esophagus.
2. **Delayed Symptoms:** Other symptoms of esophagitis may have a delayed onset, occurring hours to days after exposure to inciting factors or following initiation of therapeutic interventions. Delayed symptoms may include persistent dysphagia, chest pain, heartburn, or regurgitation, reflecting progressive mucosal inflammation, ulceration, or fibrosis in the esophagus, exacerbating symptoms over time.
3. **Nocturnal Symptoms:** Nocturnal symptoms of esophagitis, such as nighttime heartburn, regurgitation, or chest pain, may occur during periods of recumbency or following supine positioning, leading to disrupted sleep patterns, nocturnal reflux episodes, or exacerbation of symptoms overnight. Nocturnal symptoms may be more pronounced in patients with GERD or nocturnal reflux, necessitating lifestyle modifications or pharmacological interventions to improve symptom control and quality of life.
4. **Postprandial Symptoms:** Postprandial symptoms of esophagitis, such as dysphagia, retrosternal discomfort, or belching, may occur following meals or with ingestion of specific foods or beverages that

exacerbate esophageal reflux or mucosal irritation. Postprandial symptoms may be triggered by large meals, fatty foods, spicy foods, carbonated beverages, or caffeine, exacerbating reflux symptoms and impairing esophageal clearance.

5. **Intermittent Symptoms:** Intermittent symptoms of esophagitis may occur sporadically, with variable frequency and severity depending on individual triggers, dietary habits, lifestyle factors, or underlying disease activity. Intermittent symptoms may wax and wane over time, influenced by fluctuations in mucosal inflammation, reflux episodes, or response to treatment interventions, requiring ongoing monitoring and adjustment of management strategies to optimize symptom control and disease outcomes.

In summary, the clinical presentation of esophagitis varies depending on the underlying etiology, severity of mucosal injury, and patient-specific factors. Understanding the timing of symptoms is crucial for identifying potential triggers, guiding diagnostic evaluations, and implementing appropriate management strategies in patients with esophagitis of various origins. Collaborative efforts between patients, healthcare providers, and multidisciplinary teams are essential for recognizing, evaluating, and managing esophagitis to optimize outcomes and improve quality of life for affected individuals.

Diagnosis and Imaging Modalities

Accurate diagnosis of esophagitis is essential for guiding appropriate management strategies and optimizing patient outcomes. A comprehensive diagnostic approach, including clinical evaluation, endoscopic assessment, and imaging modalities, is necessary to identify underlying etiologies, assess disease severity, and detect complications associated with esophageal inflammation.

Diagnostic Modalities:

1. **Clinical Evaluation:**

Medical History: A detailed medical history is essential for identifying potential risk factors, eliciting relevant symptoms, and assessing the duration, frequency, and severity of esophageal symptoms. Inquire about past medical history, medication use, dietary habits, lifestyle factors, and occupational exposures that may predispose to esophagitis.

Symptom Assessment: Evaluate for cardinal symptoms of esophagitis, including dysphagia, odynophagia, retrosternal discomfort, heartburn, regurgitation, chest pain, or dyspeptic symptoms. Assess the timing, frequency, and severity of symptoms, as well as any associated factors that may exacerbate or alleviate symptoms.

Physical Examination: Perform a focused physical examination to assess for signs of esophageal inflammation, mucosal injury, or complications such as weight loss, malnutrition, or signs of systemic illness. Palpate for abdominal tenderness, hepatomegaly, or lymphadenopathy suggestive of underlying pathology.

2. **Endoscopic Evaluation:**

Esophagogastroduodenoscopy (EGD): EGD is the gold standard diagnostic test for evaluating esophagitis, allowing direct visualization of the esophageal mucosa, identification of mucosal abnormalities, and acquisition of biopsy specimens for histological evaluation. Endoscopic findings suggestive of esophagitis include mucosal erythema, edema, erosions, ulcerations, or strictures, which may vary in severity depending on the underlying etiology.

Biopsy Sampling: Biopsy specimens obtained during EGD are essential for confirming the diagnosis of esophagitis, assessing the degree of mucosal inflammation, and identifying specific histopathological features associated with different etiologies. Histological examination may reveal increased eosinophilic infiltration, neutrophilic inflammation, basal cell hyperplasia, or epithelial changes consistent with esophageal injury.

3. **Imaging Modalities:**

Barium Swallow: Barium swallow, or esophagography, may be performed to assess esophageal anatomy, mucosal contour, luminal narrowing, or motility disorders in patients with suspected esophagitis. Barium studies may reveal mucosal irregularities, strictures, ulcers, or filling defects suggestive of esophageal pathology.

Computed Tomography (CT) Scan: CT scan of the chest or abdomen may be indicated in patients with suspected complications of esophagitis, such as mediastinal abscess, perforation, or fistula formation. CT imaging can provide detailed anatomical information, assess for extraluminal abnormalities, and guide further management decisions in complex cases.

Magnetic Resonance Imaging (MRI): MRI may be utilized for evaluating esophageal disorders, particularly in patients with contraindications to CT or when additional soft tissue characterization is required. MRI can assess for esophageal wall thickening, luminal narrowing, or adjacent organ involvement, providing valuable diagnostic information in selected cases.

Endoscopic Ultrasound (EUS): EUS may be performed to evaluate for locoregional staging of esophageal malignancies, assess for depth of tumor invasion, lymph node involvement, or adjacent organ infiltration. EUS can provide high-resolution imaging of the esophageal wall layers, facilitating accurate staging and guiding treatment planning in patients with esophageal cancer.

Diagnostic Algorithm:

1. **Clinical Evaluation:** Obtain a comprehensive medical history, perform a physical examination, and assess for cardinal symptoms of esophagitis.
2. **Endoscopic Evaluation:** Perform EGD with biopsy sampling to visualize the esophageal mucosa, identify mucosal abnormalities, and obtain histological specimens for further evaluation.
3. **Imaging Studies:** Consider adjunctive imaging modalities such as barium swallow, CT scan, MRI, or EUS to assess for complications, evaluate for extraluminal abnormalities, or guide treatment decisions in selected cases.
4. **Multidisciplinary Collaboration:** Collaborate with gastroenterologists, radiologists, pathologists, and other specialists to interpret diagnostic findings, formulate a differential diagnosis, and develop an individualized management plan for patients with esophagitis.

In summary, accurate diagnosis of esophagitis requires a systematic approach incorporating clinical evaluation, endoscopic assessment, and imaging modalities to identify underlying etiologies, assess disease severity, and detect complications associated with esophageal inflammation. Collaboration between healthcare providers, multidisciplinary teams, and specialized diagnostic services is essential for optimizing diagnostic accuracy, guiding appropriate management strategies, and improving outcomes for patients with esophagitis.

Management Strategies and Supportive Care

Effective management of esophagitis involves a multidimensional approach aimed at alleviating symptoms, promoting mucosal healing, preventing complications, and improving overall quality of life for affected individuals. Management strategies encompass pharmacological therapy, dietary modification, lifestyle interventions, and supportive care measures tailored to the underlying etiology, severity of symptoms, and individual patient characteristics.

Pharmacological Therapy:

1. **Acid Suppression:**

Proton Pump Inhibitors (PPIs): PPIs are first-line agents for the treatment of GERD-related esophagitis, providing potent and sustained suppression of gastric acid secretion. PPIs promote mucosal healing, alleviate symptoms of heartburn and regurgitation, and reduce the risk of esophageal complications such as strictures or Barrett's esophagus.

Histamine-2 Receptor Antagonists (H2RAs): H2RAs may be used as alternative or adjunctive therapy for the management of mild to moderate esophagitis, providing reversible inhibition of gastric acid secretion and symptom relief in selected patients.

2. **Mucosal Protection:**

Sucralfate: Sucralfate forms a protective barrier over the gastric and esophageal mucosa, promoting mucosal healing and reducing the risk of ulceration or erosions in patients with reflux esophagitis or NSAID-induced injury.

Prostaglandin Analogues: Prostaglandin analogues such as misoprostol may be prescribed to enhance mucosal protection, stimulate mucus secretion, and reduce the risk of NSAID-induced gastroduodenal injury in high-risk patients.

3. **Anti-inflammatory Agents:**

Topical Steroids: Topical steroids such as swallowed fluticasone or budesonide may be used as first-line therapy for eosinophilic esophagitis (EoE), reducing esophageal inflammation, eosinophilic infiltration, and fibrotic changes in affected individuals.

4. **Antibiotics:**

Antibiotic Therapy: Antibiotic therapy may be indicated for the management of infectious esophagitis secondary to bacterial, fungal, viral, or parasitic pathogens, targeting specific causative organisms and reducing microbial burden in the esophageal lumen.

Dietary Modification:

1. **Acidic and Irritant Foods:** Advise patients to avoid acidic, spicy, or irritant foods and beverages that may exacerbate symptoms of esophagitis, such as citrus fruits, tomatoes, caffeine, alcohol, carbonated drinks, and hot spices.
2. **Dietary Triggers:** Identify and eliminate dietary triggers that may provoke esophageal symptoms, such as allergenic foods, gluten-containing grains, dairy products, or high-cholesterol foods, in patients with eosinophilic esophagitis or food sensitivities.
3. **Soft and Easily Digestible Foods:** Encourage consumption of soft, bland, and easily digestible foods that are gentle on the esophageal mucosa and facilitate swallowing in patients with dysphagia or odynophagia.
4. **Nutritional Supplementation:** Provide nutritional supplementation, enteral feeding, or parenteral

nutrition as needed to maintain adequate caloric intake, prevent malnutrition, and support mucosal healing in patients with severe or refractory esophagitis.

Lifestyle Interventions:

1. **Weight Management:** Encourage weight management strategies, including dietary modification, regular physical activity, and lifestyle changes aimed at achieving and maintaining a healthy weight in overweight or obese individuals with GERD-related esophagitis.
2. **Smoking Cessation:** Advise patients to quit smoking and avoid tobacco use, as smoking is a known risk factor for esophageal inflammation, reflux symptoms, and complications of esophagitis.
3. **Alcohol Reduction:** Limit alcohol consumption and avoid excessive intake of alcoholic beverages, as alcohol can exacerbate reflux symptoms, impair esophageal motility, and increase the risk of esophageal injury in susceptible individuals.
4. **Postural Changes:** Recommend postural changes such as elevating the head of the bed, avoiding supine positioning immediately after meals, and maintaining an upright posture during and after eating to reduce the risk of nocturnal reflux and promote esophageal clearance.

Supportive Care Measures:

1. **Symptom Management:** Provide symptomatic relief with over-the-counter antacids, alginate-based formulations, or viscous lidocaine for immediate relief of heartburn, regurgitation, or retrosternal discomfort in patients with mild to moderate symptoms of

esophagitis.
2. **Pain Management:** Administer analgesic medications such as acetaminophen, nonsteroidal anti-inflammatory drugs (NSAIDs), or opioids as needed to alleviate chest pain, dysphagia, or odynophagia associated with esophageal inflammation or mucosal injury.
3. **Hydration:** Encourage adequate hydration with water, clear fluids, or oral rehydration solutions to maintain hydration status, prevent dehydration, and facilitate mucosal healing in patients with esophagitis.
4. **Nutritional Support:** Provide nutritional counseling, dietary guidance, and meal planning assistance to ensure adequate nutrient intake, optimize nutritional status, and promote recovery in patients with esophagitis-associated malnutrition or weight loss.

In summary, effective management of esophagitis involves a comprehensive approach incorporating pharmacological therapy, dietary modification, lifestyle interventions, and supportive care measures tailored to individual patient characteristics, underlying etiologies, and severity of symptoms. Multidisciplinary collaboration between healthcare providers, gastroenterologists, dietitians, and supportive care teams is essential for optimizing treatment outcomes, preventing complications, and improving quality of life for patients with esophagitis.

CHAPTER 8: REFRACTORY ESOPHAGITIS AND COMPLICATIONS

Definition and Criteria for Refractory Disease

Refractory esophagitis refers to a challenging clinical scenario in which patients fail to achieve symptomatic relief or mucosal healing despite appropriate treatment interventions and optimization of management strategies. The definition of refractory disease varies depending on the underlying etiology, severity of symptoms, and response to therapy, necessitating a comprehensive approach to diagnosis, evaluation, and management in affected individuals.

Definition of Refractory Esophagitis:

1. **Persistent Symptoms:** Refractory esophagitis is characterized by the persistence or recurrence of esophageal symptoms despite adequate treatment with standard pharmacological therapy, dietary modification, lifestyle interventions, or endoscopic

interventions aimed at symptom control and mucosal healing.
2. **Failure to Achieve Remission:** Refractory esophagitis may occur when patients fail to achieve symptomatic remission or mucosal healing despite adherence to recommended treatment regimens, optimization of therapy, and implementation of supportive care measures tailored to individual patient needs.
3. **Duration of Symptoms:** Refractory esophagitis may be defined based on the duration and severity of symptoms, with persistent or recurrent symptoms lasting beyond the expected timeframe for resolution or improvement with standard treatment approaches.

Criteria for Refractory Disease:

1. **Clinical Symptoms:**

Persistent Dysphagia: Refractory esophagitis may be characterized by persistent or recurrent dysphagia despite adequate acid suppression therapy, dietary modification, or endoscopic interventions aimed at improving esophageal patency and swallowing function.

Refractory Heartburn: Refractory esophagitis may manifest as refractory heartburn or regurgitation, with ongoing or recurrent symptoms of gastroesophageal reflux despite maximal acid suppression therapy and lifestyle modifications.

Treatment-Resistant Chest Pain: Refractory esophagitis may present with treatment-resistant chest pain or retrosternal discomfort, persisting despite empiric therapy with proton pump inhibitors (PPIs), antacids, or analgesic medications.

2. **Endoscopic Findings:**

Persistent Mucosal Erosions or Ulcerations: Refractory esophagitis may be confirmed by endoscopic evaluation demonstrating persistent mucosal erosions, ulcerations, or inflammatory changes despite ongoing treatment with acid-suppressive therapy or mucosal protection agents.

Failure to Achieve Mucosal Healing: Refractory esophagitis may be defined based on failure to achieve mucosal healing or resolution of endoscopic abnormalities despite prolonged treatment duration and optimization of therapeutic interventions.

   3. **Histological Evaluation:**

Persistent Inflammation: Refractory esophagitis may be supported by histological evaluation of esophageal biopsy specimens demonstrating persistent inflammation, eosinophilic infiltration, or epithelial changes consistent with ongoing mucosal injury despite treatment with anti-inflammatory agents or steroid therapy.

   4. **Objective Testing:**

Recurrent Abnormal pH Monitoring: Refractory esophagitis may be confirmed by recurrent abnormal findings on ambulatory esophageal pH monitoring, demonstrating persistent acid reflux, nonacid reflux, or weakly acidic reflux events despite maximal acid suppression therapy.

Refractory Impedance Testing: Refractory esophagitis may be identified by refractory impedance testing demonstrating persistent esophageal reflux, bolus clearance abnormalities, or hypersensitivity to reflux events despite treatment optimization and lifestyle modifications.

Management Challenges:

   1. **Identification of Underlying Etiology:** Refractory esophagitis requires a systematic approach to identify potential underlying etiologies, including GERD, eosinophilic esophagitis, infectious esophagitis, medication-induced injury, or functional esophageal disorders, which may require targeted diagnostic evaluations and tailored management strategies.
   2. **Multimodal Treatment Approaches:** Refractory

esophagitis may necessitate multimodal treatment approaches incorporating pharmacological therapy, dietary modification, lifestyle interventions, endoscopic interventions, or surgical options tailored to individual patient characteristics, disease severity, and underlying etiologies.
3. **Specialized Referral:** Refractory esophagitis may require specialized referral to tertiary care centers, academic medical centers, or specialized gastroenterology practices with expertise in the diagnosis and management of complex esophageal disorders, facilitating access to advanced diagnostic modalities, novel therapeutic interventions, and multidisciplinary care teams.

In summary, refractory esophagitis represents a challenging clinical scenario characterized by persistent or recurrent symptoms and mucosal abnormalities despite appropriate treatment interventions. The definition and criteria for refractory disease emphasize the importance of thorough diagnostic evaluation, optimization of management strategies, and consideration of underlying etiologies to improve outcomes and quality of life for affected individuals. Collaborative efforts between patients, healthcare providers, and multidisciplinary teams are essential for recognizing, evaluating, and managing refractory esophagitis effectively.

Underlying Causes and Contributing Factors

Refractory esophagitis poses a diagnostic and therapeutic challenge, often requiring a comprehensive evaluation to identify underlying causes and contributing factors that may contribute to treatment failure or persistent symptoms. Understanding the diverse etiologies and potential mechanisms involved in refractory disease is essential for guiding targeted interventions and optimizing management strategies in affected individuals.

Underlying Causes:

1. **Gastroesophageal Reflux Disease (GERD):**

Esophageal Hypersensitivity: Patients with GERD-related esophagitis may exhibit esophageal hypersensitivity, characterized by heightened perception of reflux events, increased visceral sensitivity, or abnormal pain processing mechanisms, contributing to persistent symptoms despite acid suppression therapy.

Reflux Hypoallergenic Diet: Some individuals with refractory GERD may have underlying food allergies or sensitivities contributing to esophageal inflammation, mucosal injury, or dysmotility, necessitating evaluation for food triggers and implementation of a reflux hypoallergenic diet to achieve symptom control and mucosal healing.

2. **Eosinophilic Esophagitis (EoE):**

Allergic Mechanisms: EoE is an immune-mediated disorder characterized by eosinophilic inflammation of the esophagus, triggered by allergen exposure, environmental factors, or genetic predisposition. Refractory EoE may result from ongoing allergen exposure, dietary triggers, or inadequate response to corticosteroid therapy, necessitating targeted elimination diets, elemental formulas, or biologic agents for disease control.

Treatment-Resistant Fibrosis: Some patients with refractory EoE may develop treatment-resistant fibrosis, strictures, or luminal narrowing in the esophagus, requiring endoscopic dilation, stent placement, or surgical intervention to alleviate dysphagia and improve esophageal patency.

3. **Infectious Esophagitis:**

Antifungal Resistance: Patients with infectious esophagitis, particularly candidal esophagitis, may develop antifungal resistance, treatment failure, or recurrent infections due to underlying immunocompromised states, mucosal disruption, or biofilm formation, necessitating alternative antifungal agents, combination therapy, or extended treatment durations for infection control.

Antibiotic Resistance: Infectious esophagitis caused by bacterial, viral, or parasitic pathogens may exhibit antibiotic resistance, treatment failure, or recurrent infections due to microbial virulence factors, host immune responses, or bacterial biofilm formation, requiring targeted antimicrobial therapy guided by susceptibility testing or molecular diagnostics.

4. **Medication-Induced Esophagitis:**

Drug Interactions: Refractory esophagitis may result from medication-induced injury, drug interactions, or adverse effects of pharmacological agents such as nonsteroidal anti-inflammatory drugs (NSAIDs), bisphosphonates, potassium supplements, or oral medications with esophageal irritant properties, necessitating medication reconciliation, dose adjustments, or alternative formulations to minimize mucosal injury and improve tolerability.

Chemical Esophagitis: Chemical esophagitis may occur due to accidental ingestion of corrosive substances, caustic medications, or chemical irritants, leading to acute mucosal injury, ulceration, or strictures in the esophagus, which may require emergent endoscopic evaluation, supportive care measures, or surgical intervention to prevent complications and promote healing.

Contributing Factors:

1. **Obesity and Metabolic Syndrome:** Obesity and metabolic syndrome are risk factors for GERD-related esophagitis, hiatal hernia, and impaired esophageal

motility, contributing to treatment resistance, recurrent symptoms, and complications of esophagitis in affected individuals.

2. **Dietary Habits:** Dietary factors such as high-fat foods, spicy foods, caffeine, alcohol, or carbonated beverages may exacerbate reflux symptoms, trigger esophageal inflammation, or delay mucosal healing in patients with esophagitis, necessitating dietary modification, nutritional counseling, or elimination diets to achieve symptom control and optimize treatment outcomes.

3. **Smoking and Alcohol Use:** Tobacco smoking and alcohol consumption are known risk factors for GERD-related esophagitis, Barrett's esophagus, and esophageal adenocarcinoma, exacerbating mucosal injury, promoting inflammation, and impairing esophageal clearance mechanisms, which may contribute to treatment resistance and disease progression in affected individuals.

4. **Psychosocial Factors:** Psychosocial factors such as stress, anxiety, depression, or somatization disorders may influence esophageal symptoms, visceral hypersensitivity, or treatment adherence in patients with refractory esophagitis, highlighting the importance of psychosocial support, behavioral interventions, or cognitive-behavioral therapy as adjunctive measures in comprehensive management strategies.

Diagnostic Challenges:

1. **Underlying Etiology:** Identifying the underlying etiology of refractory esophagitis requires a systematic approach, including thorough clinical evaluation, endoscopic assessment, histological evaluation, and targeted diagnostic testing to differentiate between GERD, EoE, infectious esophagitis, medication-

induced injury, or other contributing factors.

2. **Diagnostic Testing:** Refractory esophagitis may necessitate advanced diagnostic testing such as ambulatory esophageal pH monitoring, esophageal manometry, impedance testing, allergen-specific IgE testing, or molecular diagnostics to characterize reflux patterns, assess esophageal motility, identify food triggers, or detect underlying immune-mediated mechanisms contributing to treatment resistance.

Management Strategies:

1. **Targeted Therapy:** Tailoring treatment strategies to the underlying etiology and contributing factors of refractory esophagitis is essential for optimizing treatment outcomes and achieving symptomatic relief. Targeted therapies may include elimination diets, biologic agents, immune-modulating agents, or alternative pharmacological agents based on individual patient characteristics and disease severity.

2. **Multidisciplinary Collaboration:** Collaborative efforts between gastroenterologists, allergists, dietitians, pharmacists, psychologists, and other specialists are essential for managing refractory esophagitis effectively, integrating comprehensive diagnostic evaluations, personalized treatment plans, and supportive care measures to address the diverse needs of affected individuals.

In summary, refractory esophagitis encompasses a spectrum of challenging clinical scenarios characterized by persistent symptoms, mucosal abnormalities, or treatment resistance despite appropriate interventions. Understanding the diverse etiologies, underlying mechanisms, and contributing factors involved in refractory disease is essential for guiding targeted diagnostic evaluations, optimizing treatment strategies, and improving outcomes for affected individuals. Collaborative efforts between patients, healthcare providers, and multidisciplinary teams are essential for recognizing, evaluating, and managing refractory esophagitis comprehensively.

Complications: Strictures, Barrett's Esophagus, and Dysplasia

Refractory esophagitis poses a significant risk of complications, including the development of strictures, Barrett's esophagus, and dysplasia, which may necessitate additional interventions, surveillance, and management strategies to mitigate risks and optimize outcomes in affected individuals.

Complications of Refractory Esophagitis:

1. **Esophageal Strictures:**

Definition: Esophageal strictures are characterized by luminal narrowing, fibrosis, or scarring in the esophagus, resulting from chronic inflammation, mucosal injury, or healing processes in response to reflux esophagitis, eosinophilic esophagitis, or other underlying etiologies.

Clinical Manifestations: Esophageal strictures may present with dysphagia, odynophagia, or food impaction, reflecting impaired bolus transit, luminal obstruction, or mechanical obstruction secondary to luminal narrowing.

Diagnostic Evaluation: Esophageal strictures are diagnosed based on endoscopic evaluation demonstrating luminal narrowing, mucosal irregularities, or circumferential scarring in the esophagus, which may require endoscopic dilation, esophageal stent placement, or surgical intervention for symptomatic relief and restoration of esophageal patency.

2. Barrett's Esophagus:

Definition: Barrett's esophagus is a premalignant condition characterized by metaplastic changes in the esophageal epithelium, with replacement of normal squamous epithelium by specialized intestinal metaplasia in response to chronic gastroesophageal reflux or esophagitis.

Clinical Significance: Barrett's esophagus is associated with an increased risk of esophageal adenocarcinoma, highlighting the importance of surveillance endoscopy, histological evaluation, and risk stratification in affected individuals.

Diagnostic Evaluation: Barrett's esophagus is diagnosed based on endoscopic evaluation demonstrating columnar-lined epithelium with intestinal metaplasia in the distal esophagus, which may require endoscopic surveillance, biopsy sampling, or advanced imaging modalities for early detection and management of dysplastic changes.

3. Dysplasia and Neoplastic Progression:

Definition: Dysplasia refers to the presence of abnormal cellular changes, characterized by cellular atypia, architectural distortion, or increased mitotic activity in the esophageal epithelium, which may progress to invasive neoplasia if left untreated.

Clinical Significance: Dysplasia in Barrett's esophagus is a key predictor of neoplastic progression, with low-grade dysplasia carrying a lower risk of progression compared to high-grade dysplasia, necessitating close surveillance, histological evaluation, and risk stratification for appropriate management decisions.

Diagnostic Evaluation: Dysplasia in Barrett's esophagus is diagnosed based on histological evaluation of biopsy specimens obtained during surveillance endoscopy, which may require advanced imaging modalities, molecular biomarkers, or endoscopic resection techniques for accurate staging and risk assessment.

Management Strategies:

1. **Endoscopic Dilation:** Esophageal strictures may be managed with endoscopic dilation techniques, balloon dilation, or bougie dilators to improve luminal patency, alleviate dysphagia, and prevent recurrent food impaction in affected individuals.
2. **Endoscopic Mucosal Resection (EMR):** Barrett's esophagus with dysplasia may be managed with endoscopic mucosal resection techniques, ablative therapies, or endoscopic submucosal dissection for removal of dysplastic or neoplastic lesions, reducing the risk of progression to invasive carcinoma.
3. **Radiofrequency Ablation (RFA):** Barrett's esophagus with low-grade dysplasia or early neoplasia may be treated with radiofrequency ablation, thermal energy delivery, or cryotherapy to eliminate metaplastic or dysplastic epithelium, reducing the risk of neoplastic progression and improving long-term outcomes.
4. **Surgical Intervention:** Refractory esophagitis with complications such as strictures, Barrett's esophagus, or dysplasia may require surgical intervention, esophagectomy, or minimally invasive procedures to alleviate symptoms, prevent malignant transformation, and improve overall survival in selected cases.

Surveillance and Follow-Up:

1. **Endoscopic Surveillance:** Patients with refractory esophagitis, strictures, Barrett's esophagus, or dysplasia require regular endoscopic surveillance with biopsy sampling to monitor disease progression, assess for complications, and guide management decisions based on histological evaluation and risk

stratification.
2. **Interval Endoscopy:** Surveillance endoscopy intervals may vary depending on the presence of dysplasia, degree of mucosal abnormalities, and individual patient characteristics, with more frequent surveillance recommended for high-risk lesions or advanced neoplasia requiring closer monitoring and early intervention.

In summary, refractory esophagitis is associated with a spectrum of complications, including strictures, Barrett's esophagus, and dysplasia, which necessitate vigilant surveillance, targeted interventions, and multidisciplinary management strategies to mitigate risks, optimize outcomes, and improve long-term prognosis in affected individuals. Collaborative efforts between gastroenterologists, surgeons, pathologists, and supportive care teams are essential for recognizing, evaluating, and managing complications of refractory esophagitis comprehensively.

Treatment Challenges and Novel Therapeutic Options

Refractory esophagitis presents significant treatment challenges due to the complex interplay of underlying etiologies, contributing factors, and pathophysiological mechanisms involved in disease pathogenesis. Despite advances in diagnostic modalities and therapeutic interventions, some patients continue to experience persistent symptoms, mucosal abnormalities, or complications that require innovative approaches and novel therapeutic options to improve outcomes and quality of life.

Treatment Challenges:

1. **Multifactorial Etiology:** Refractory esophagitis often arises from a multifactorial interplay of underlying etiologies, including gastroesophageal reflux disease (GERD), eosinophilic esophagitis (EoE), infectious esophagitis, medication-induced injury, or functional esophageal disorders, necessitating a comprehensive diagnostic evaluation and targeted treatment approach to address individual patient needs.
2. **Treatment Resistance:** Some patients with refractory esophagitis exhibit treatment resistance or inadequate response to standard pharmacological therapy, dietary modification, lifestyle interventions, or endoscopic interventions, highlighting the need for alternative treatment strategies, adjunctive therapies, or combination regimens to achieve symptomatic relief and mucosal healing.
3. **Complications and Comorbidities:** Refractory esophagitis is associated with a spectrum of complications, including strictures, Barrett's esophagus, dysplasia, or esophageal adenocarcinoma, which may necessitate additional interventions, surveillance, or management strategies to mitigate risks and optimize outcomes in affected individuals with complex medical histories or comorbid conditions.
4. **Psychosocial Factors:** Psychosocial factors such as stress, anxiety, depression, or somatization disorders may influence esophageal symptoms, visceral hypersensitivity, treatment adherence, or response to therapy in patients with refractory esophagitis, underscoring the importance of psychosocial support, behavioral interventions, or cognitive-behavioral therapy as adjunctive measures in comprehensive

management strategies.

Novel Therapeutic Options:

1. **Biologic Agents:**

Anti-inflammatory Biologics: Biologic agents targeting specific inflammatory pathways implicated in esophageal inflammation, fibrosis, or dysmotility may offer novel therapeutic options for refractory esophagitis, including anti-IL-5 antibodies (e.g., mepolizumab), anti-IL-13 antibodies (e.g., dupilumab), or anti-TNF-alpha agents (e.g., infliximab), which have shown promise in clinical trials for the treatment of EoE or refractory GERD.

2. **Immunomodulatory Therapies:**

Immunosuppressive Agents: Immunomodulatory agents such as azathioprine, 6-mercaptopurine, or methotrexate may be considered for the management of refractory esophagitis associated with autoimmune disorders, connective tissue diseases, or immunodeficiency states, targeting aberrant immune responses, cytokine dysregulation, or lymphocyte activation implicated in disease pathogenesis.

3. **Targeted Therapies:**

Molecular Targeted Agents: Molecular targeted therapies targeting specific molecular pathways implicated in esophageal carcinogenesis, angiogenesis, or tumor growth may offer novel treatment options for refractory esophagitis with dysplasia or neoplastic progression, including tyrosine kinase inhibitors (e.g., imatinib, dasatinib), vascular endothelial growth factor (VEGF) inhibitors (e.g., bevacizumab), or epidermal growth factor receptor (EGFR) inhibitors (e.g., cetuximab), which have shown potential in preclinical studies or early-phase clinical trials.

4. **Advanced Endoscopic Techniques:**

Endoscopic Submucosal Dissection (ESD): Endoscopic submucosal dissection techniques allow en bloc resection of early neoplastic lesions, high-grade dysplasia, or intramucosal carcinomas in Barrett's esophagus, offering curative treatment options for selected patients with refractory esophagitis and superficial neoplastic lesions not amenable to conventional endoscopic resection techniques.

5. **Implantable Devices:**

Anti-reflux Devices: Implantable anti-reflux devices such as the LINX Reflux Management System or magnetic sphincter augmentation devices may offer novel treatment options for refractory GERD, providing mechanical reinforcement of the lower esophageal sphincter, reduction of transient lower esophageal sphincter relaxations, and improvement of reflux control in selected patients with persistent symptoms despite maximal acid suppression therapy or lifestyle modifications.

Clinical Trials and Research Directions:

1. **Biomarker Discovery:** Identification of novel biomarkers, molecular signatures, or genetic markers associated with refractory esophagitis may facilitate early diagnosis, risk stratification, treatment response prediction, and personalized therapeutic interventions in affected individuals, guiding clinical decision-making and optimizing treatment outcomes.
2. **Precision Medicine:** Advancements in precision medicine, pharmacogenomics, or targeted therapies may enable individualized treatment approaches tailored to specific patient characteristics, disease phenotypes, or underlying molecular pathways implicated in refractory esophagitis, optimizing therapeutic efficacy, minimizing adverse effects, and improving patient adherence.
3. **Regenerative Medicine:** Exploration of regenerative medicine approaches, tissue engineering techniques, or stem cell therapies may offer innovative treatment

options for refractory esophagitis, promoting mucosal regeneration, tissue repair, or functional restoration in patients with severe mucosal injury, strictures, or dysmotility disorders not amenable to conventional therapies.

In summary, refractory esophagitis presents significant treatment challenges necessitating innovative approaches and novel therapeutic options to improve outcomes, alleviate symptoms, and prevent complications in affected individuals. Ongoing research efforts, clinical trials, and advancements in precision medicine hold promise for the development of targeted interventions, personalized treatment strategies, and improved management approaches for refractory esophagitis in the future.

CHAPTER 9: DIAGNOSTIC APPROACHES IN ESOPHAGITIS

History and Physical Examination

The cornerstone of diagnosing esophagitis lies in a comprehensive history-taking and a meticulous physical examination. This initial step provides crucial insights into the patient's symptoms, medical history, and potential risk factors, aiding in the formulation of an accurate diagnostic and management plan.

History:

1. **Presenting Symptoms:**

Dysphagia: Inquire about difficulty swallowing, including solids or liquids, and any associated pain or discomfort.

Heartburn: Assess the presence and severity of retrosternal burning sensations or acid regurgitation, especially after meals or when lying down.

Odynophagia: Explore for painful swallowing, which may indicate mucosal inflammation or injury.

Regurgitation: Ask about the involuntary return of food or gastric contents into the mouth, often accompanied by a sour taste.

Chest Pain: Evaluate for chest discomfort, potentially confused with cardiac issues, especially if related to swallowing or meal ingestion.

Weight Loss: Inquire about unintended weight loss, which could be indicative of severe esophageal disease or obstructive processes.

2. **Symptom Duration and Progression:**

Determine when symptoms first appeared, how they have evolved over time, and if any exacerbating or alleviating factors are identified.

3. **Medical History:**

GERD: Assess for a history of gastroesophageal reflux disease (GERD), including previous diagnoses, treatments, and responses to medications.

Medication Use: Document any current medications, particularly NSAIDs, bisphosphonates, or potassium supplements, which can contribute to esophageal irritation.

Allergies and Dietary Habits: Explore potential food allergies, intolerances, or dietary patterns that may exacerbate symptoms.

Medical Conditions: Identify comorbidities such as autoimmune diseases, connective tissue disorders, or immunocompromised states that could predispose to esophageal inflammation or infection.

4. **Lifestyle Factors:**

Diet and Habits: Investigate dietary habits, alcohol consumption, tobacco use, and caffeine intake, as they can influence esophageal function and exacerbate symptoms.

Physical Activity: Assess the patient's level of physical activity and its potential impact on gastrointestinal motility and reflux symptoms.

5. **Family History:**

Esophageal Disorders: Inquire about a family history of esophageal disorders, including esophagitis, Barrett's esophagus, or esophageal cancer, which may indicate genetic predispositions or shared environmental factors.

Physical Examination:

1. **General Appearance:**

Evaluate the patient's general demeanor, nutritional status, and hydration level, noting any signs of distress or malnutrition.

2. **Vital Signs:**

Measure vital signs, including blood pressure, heart rate, respiratory rate, and temperature, to assess for signs of systemic illness or dehydration.

3. **Oral Cavity and Neck:**

Inspect the oral cavity for signs of mucosal inflammation, lesions, or thrush, which may indicate oropharyngeal involvement.

Palpate the neck for lymphadenopathy, masses, or thyromegaly, which could suggest infectious, inflammatory, or neoplastic processes.

4. **Chest and Abdomen:**

Auscultate the chest for abnormal breath sounds and percuss for dullness, which may suggest underlying pulmonary or pleural pathology.

Palpate the abdomen for tenderness, organomegaly, or masses, assessing for signs of intra-abdominal pathology or extrinsic compression of the esophagus.

5. **Cardiovascular and Respiratory Systems:**

Listen for murmurs, irregular heart sounds, or crackles on lung auscultation, considering cardiac and respiratory causes of chest pain or dysphagia.

6. **Neurological Examination:**

Perform a focused neurological examination to assess cranial nerve function, motor strength, and sensation, particularly if dysphagia is present.

By gathering a detailed history and conducting a thorough physical examination, healthcare providers can establish a foundation for further diagnostic evaluation and tailor management strategies to address the specific needs of patients with esophagitis.

Endoscopic Evaluation: Techniques and Findings

Endoscopic evaluation is a cornerstone in diagnosing esophagitis, offering direct visualization of the esophageal mucosa and providing valuable information about mucosal integrity, inflammation, and structural abnormalities. Various endoscopic techniques and findings play crucial roles in identifying and characterizing esophageal pathology.

Techniques:

1. **Upper Endoscopy (Esophagogastroduodenoscopy - EGD):**

Upper endoscopy is the gold standard for evaluating esophageal pathology.

A flexible endoscope is inserted through the mouth and advanced into the esophagus, allowing visualization of the esophageal mucosa, gastroesophageal junction (GEJ), and proximal stomach.

High-definition endoscopes provide superior image quality,

enabling detailed examination of mucosal features and abnormalities.

Endoscopic retrograde cholangiopancreatography (ERCP) or endoscopic ultrasound (EUS) may be adjunctive procedures to evaluate the biliary or pancreatic ducts or assess the depth of esophageal lesions, respectively.

2. Virtual Chromoendoscopy:

Virtual chromoendoscopy techniques, such as narrow-band imaging (NBI) or i-Scan, enhance mucosal visualization by highlighting subtle vascular patterns and mucosal surface characteristics.

These techniques aid in detecting subtle mucosal changes, distinguishing between benign and malignant lesions, and guiding targeted biopsies.

3. Magnification Endoscopy:

Magnification endoscopy allows for enhanced visualization of mucosal details and microvascular patterns.

It aids in the characterization of mucosal lesions, assessment of mucosal architecture, and identification of early neoplastic changes.

Advanced imaging modalities, such as magnification with NBI or magnification with optical coherence tomography (OCT), further improve diagnostic accuracy.

4. Endoscopic Ultrasound (EUS):

EUS utilizes high-frequency ultrasound waves to evaluate the layers of the esophageal wall and adjacent structures.

It provides detailed imaging of the mucosa, submucosa, muscularis propria, and surrounding lymph nodes, aiding in the staging of esophageal cancer and assessment of lesion depth.

Findings:

1. Esophagitis Grading:

The Los Angeles Classification system categorizes esophagitis based on endoscopic findings into grades ranging from A to D, reflecting the severity of mucosal injury and erosions.

Grade A: Isolated mucosal erythema or edema.
Grade B: Mucosal breaks less than 5 mm in length.
Grade C: Mucosal breaks more than 5 mm in length, but not continuous between mucosal folds.
Grade D: Continuous mucosal breaks involving at least 75% of the esophageal circumference.

2. **Mucosal Abnormalities:**

Erythema: Redness or inflammation of the esophageal mucosa, suggestive of acute inflammation or mucosal injury.
Erosions: Superficial defects or breaks in the mucosal surface, indicative of mucosal damage or ulceration.
Ulcers: Deeper defects in the mucosa with loss of tissue integrity, often associated with more severe inflammation or injury.
Strictures: Luminal narrowing or strictures resulting from chronic inflammation, fibrosis, or scarring of the esophageal wall.

3. **Barrett's Esophagus:**

Barrett's esophagus is characterized by the replacement of normal squamous epithelium with columnar epithelium containing intestinal metaplasia.
Endoscopic findings include salmon-colored mucosa with visible vascular markings, irregular Z-line, or tongues of columnar epithelium extending proximally from the GEJ.

4. **Neoplastic Lesions:**

Endoscopic features of esophageal neoplasms vary depending on the subtype (e.g., squamous cell carcinoma, adenocarcinoma).
Squamous cell carcinoma may present as exophytic or ulcerated lesions with irregular borders and friable mucosa.
Adenocarcinoma often manifests as raised or nodular masses, irregular mucosal surfaces, or strictures with luminal narrowing.

Endoscopic evaluation provides crucial information for diagnosing esophagitis, assessing disease severity, guiding treatment decisions, and monitoring disease progression. Combining advanced endoscopic techniques with meticulous examination skills enhances diagnostic accuracy and improves patient outcomes.

Histopathological Assessment and Biopsy Interpretation

Histopathological assessment of esophageal tissue obtained through endoscopic biopsies plays a critical role in confirming the diagnosis of esophagitis, identifying underlying etiologies, and guiding treatment decisions. Interpretation of biopsy findings requires careful examination of histological features, inflammatory changes, and specific patterns of tissue injury.

Histopathological Techniques:

1. **Biopsy Collection:**

Biopsies are obtained during upper endoscopy using forceps passed through the endoscope.

Multiple biopsy samples are typically taken from different locations along the esophagus to ensure representative sampling of the mucosa.

2. **Tissue Processing:**

Biopsy specimens are fixed in formalin and processed in the histology laboratory.

After embedding in paraffin wax, thin sections of tissue are cut and stained with hematoxylin and eosin (H&E) for routine histological examination.

3. **Special Stains and Immunohistochemistry:**

Special stains, such as periodic acid-Schiff (PAS) or Giemsa, may be used to highlight specific tissue components or microorganisms.

Immunohistochemical staining techniques can identify specific cell types, inflammatory markers, or tissue antigens, aiding in the diagnosis of certain esophageal disorders.

Biopsy Interpretation:

1. **Inflammatory Changes:**

Neutrophilic Infiltrate: Presence of neutrophils within the epithelium and lamina propria suggests acute inflammation, often seen in reflux esophagitis or infectious esophagitis.

Lymphocytic Infiltrate: Predominance of lymphocytes in the lamina propria may indicate chronic inflammation, as seen in eosinophilic esophagitis or autoimmune disorders.

2. **Mucosal Injury:**

Erosions and Ulcers: Loss of surface epithelium with exposed lamina propria suggests mucosal injury or ulceration, commonly observed in reflux esophagitis, infectious esophagitis, or medication-induced injury.

Basal Cell Hyperplasia: Thickening of the basal layer of squamous epithelium, often accompanied by elongation of papillae, is a nonspecific response to mucosal injury or inflammation.

3. **Eosinophilic Infiltrate:**

Increased eosinophils within the epithelium or lamina propria (>15 eosinophils per high-power field) are characteristic of eosinophilic esophagitis, an immune-mediated disorder associated with allergic reactions or food sensitivities.

4. **Epithelial Changes:**

Squamous Cell Changes: Dysplastic changes in squamous epithelium, including cellular atypia, loss of polarity, or architectural distortion, may indicate premalignant lesions or squamous cell carcinoma.

5. **Microbial Infections:**

Fungal Elements: Identification of fungal hyphae, yeast forms, or pseudohyphae within the epithelium or mucous glands suggests candidiasis or fungal esophagitis, often associated with immunocompromised states or antibiotic use.

Viral Inclusions: Presence of viral cytopathic changes, intranuclear or intracytoplasmic inclusions, may indicate viral infections such as herpes simplex virus (HSV) or cytomegalovirus (CMV) esophagitis, commonly seen in immunocompromised individuals.

6. **Submucosal Changes:**

Fibrosis and Granulation Tissue: Deposition of collagen fibers, fibroblasts, or inflammatory cells within the submucosa suggests chronic inflammation, scarring, or healing processes associated with long-standing esophagitis or strictures.

Diagnostic Considerations:

1. **Correlation with Clinical Findings:**

Histopathological findings should be interpreted in conjunction with clinical history, endoscopic findings, and radiological studies to establish a comprehensive diagnosis and guide management decisions.

2. **Differential Diagnosis:**

Consideration of differential diagnoses, including infectious, inflammatory, allergic, autoimmune, or neoplastic etiologies, is essential for accurate diagnosis and appropriate treatment selection.

3. **Multidisciplinary Collaboration:**

Collaboration between gastroenterologists, pathologists, and other specialists facilitates accurate diagnosis, optimal patient management, and comprehensive care for individuals with esophageal disorders.

Histopathological assessment of esophageal biopsies provides valuable diagnostic information and guides therapeutic interventions in patients with esophagitis. Understanding the histological features and interpreting biopsy findings in the context of clinical presentation are essential for accurate diagnosis and effective management of esophageal diseases.

Ancillary Testing: Esophageal pH Monitoring, Manometry, and Imaging

In addition to endoscopic evaluation and histopathological assessment, ancillary testing plays a crucial role in the comprehensive evaluation of esophagitis, providing valuable information about esophageal function, acid exposure, motility disorders, and anatomical abnormalities. Esophageal pH monitoring, manometry, and imaging modalities are commonly employed to complement clinical assessment and guide management decisions.

Esophageal pH Monitoring:

1. **Ambulatory Esophageal pH Monitoring:**

Ambulatory pH monitoring measures the frequency, duration, and extent of esophageal acid exposure over a defined period (typically 24 to 48 hours).

A pH probe is placed in the distal esophagus through the nose or mouth and connected to a portable data logger worn by the patient.

pH monitoring helps assess the presence and severity of gastroesophageal reflux, characterize reflux patterns (acidic vs. non-acidic), and correlate symptoms with reflux events.

Parameters evaluated include DeMeester score, total percentage time pH < 4, number of reflux episodes, and symptom association with reflux events (SI or symptom index).

2. **Wireless pH Capsule:**

Wireless pH capsules are ingestible devices that transmit pH data from the esophagus to an external receiver over 48 to 96 hours.

Capsule-based pH monitoring offers the advantage of longer recording periods, improved patient comfort, and fewer technical limitations compared to traditional catheter-based pH probes.

Esophageal Manometry:

1. **High-Resolution Esophageal Manometry (HRM):**

HRM is a sophisticated technique that assesses esophageal motility and coordination of peristalsis using pressure sensors placed along the length of a catheter.

HRM provides detailed information about esophageal function, including resting pressure, peristaltic contractions, lower esophageal sphincter (LES) pressure, and coordination between the swallowing phases.

Metrics such as distal contractile integral (DCI), integrated relaxation pressure (IRP), and distal latency aid in diagnosing motility disorders such as achalasia, esophageal spasm, or ineffective esophageal motility (IEM).

Imaging Modalities:

1. **Barium Esophagram:**

Barium esophagram, or upper gastrointestinal (UGI) series, is a fluoroscopic imaging study that evaluates esophageal anatomy, function, and luminal patency.

Barium swallow allows visualization of mucosal irregularities, strictures, diverticula, hiatal hernias, and motility disorders such as achalasia or diffuse esophageal spasm.

2. **Computed Tomography (CT) Scan:**

CT imaging may be utilized to assess for extraluminal complications of esophagitis, including mediastinal abscesses, perforation, or malignant infiltration of adjacent structures.

CT angiography (CTA) can detect vascular anomalies, pseudoaneurysms, or arterioesophageal fistulas associated with severe esophagitis or erosive complications.

3. **Magnetic Resonance Imaging (MRI):**

MRI may be employed for assessing esophageal anatomy, evaluating luminal strictures, or characterizing soft tissue lesions.

Functional MRI (fMRI) techniques can provide dynamic assessment of esophageal motility and peristalsis, complementing manometric findings.

Multimodal Approach:

1. **Integration of Findings:**

Combining information from endoscopic, histological, pH monitoring, manometric, and imaging studies allows for a comprehensive assessment of esophageal pathology and functional abnormalities.

Multimodal evaluation aids in identifying underlying etiologies, stratifying disease severity, and tailoring individualized treatment plans for patients with esophagitis.

2. **Diagnostic Algorithm:**

A stepwise diagnostic algorithm incorporating clinical evaluation, endoscopic findings, and ancillary testing helps guide the diagnostic workup and management of esophageal disorders, optimizing patient care and outcomes.

Ancillary testing, including esophageal pH monitoring, manometry, and imaging modalities, complements clinical evaluation and aids in the diagnosis, characterization, and management of esophagitis. Integrating findings from multiple diagnostic modalities allows for a comprehensive understanding of esophageal function, motility, and anatomical abnormalities, facilitating targeted interventions and personalized treatment approaches for affected individuals.

CHAPTER 10: PHARMACOLOGICAL MANAGEMENT OF ESOPHAGITIS

Treatment of Esophagitis

Acid-Suppressive Therapy: Proton Pump Inhibitors and H2-Receptor Antagonists

Acid-suppressive therapy is the cornerstone of treatment for esophagitis, aimed at reducing gastric acid secretion, alleviating symptoms, promoting mucosal healing, and preventing disease recurrence. Proton pump inhibitors (PPIs) and H2-receptor antagonists (H2RAs) are the mainstays of acid suppression, offering effective symptom relief and mucosal protection in various forms of esophagitis.

Proton Pump Inhibitors (PPIs):

1. **Mechanism of Action:**

PPIs irreversibly inhibit the H+/K+-ATPase proton pump on parietal cells, thereby suppressing gastric acid secretion. By inhibiting acid production, PPIs raise the gastric pH, reducing the acidity of gastric contents and minimizing acid reflux into the esophagus.

2. Efficacy in Esophagitis:

PPIs are highly effective in treating erosive esophagitis, healing mucosal erosions, and relieving symptoms such as heartburn, regurgitation, and dysphagia.

They provide superior healing rates compared to H2RAs and are considered first-line therapy for moderate to severe esophagitis.

3. Dosage and Administration:

Standard doses of PPIs (e.g., omeprazole, lansoprazole, pantoprazole, esomeprazole) are typically administered once daily, preferably in the morning before breakfast.

Higher doses or twice-daily dosing may be required for refractory cases or severe esophagitis.

4. Duration of Therapy:

The duration of PPI therapy depends on the severity of esophagitis, underlying etiology, and individual patient factors. Short-term courses (4-8 weeks) are usually sufficient to achieve mucosal healing in uncomplicated cases, while maintenance therapy may be necessary for chronic or recurrent esophagitis.

5. Adverse Effects:

PPIs are generally well-tolerated, with the most common side effects being mild and transient (e.g., headache, abdominal pain, diarrhea).

Long-term use of PPIs has been associated with potential risks, including increased susceptibility to gastrointestinal infections, micronutrient deficiencies (e.g., vitamin B12, magnesium), and bone fractures.

H2-Receptor Antagonists (H2RAs):

1. Mechanism of Action:

H2RAs competitively block histamine H2 receptors on parietal cells, reducing histamine-mediated stimulation of gastric acid secretion.

While less potent than PPIs, H2RAs effectively reduce basal and meal-stimulated acid secretion, providing symptomatic relief in mild to moderate cases of esophagitis.

2. **Efficacy in Esophagitis:**

H2RAs are less effective than PPIs in healing erosive esophagitis but may be considered as alternative or adjunctive therapy in mild cases or for symptom management.

They provide symptomatic relief from heartburn and regurgitation but may be insufficient for complete mucosal healing in severe esophagitis.

3. **Dosage and Administration:**

Standard doses of H2RAs (e.g., ranitidine, famotidine, cimetidine) are typically administered orally, either once or twice daily, with or without food.

Intravenous formulations may be used for hospitalized patients unable to tolerate oral medications.

4. **Duration of Therapy:**

H2RAs are often used for short-term symptomatic relief in acute esophagitis or as on-demand therapy for mild symptoms.

They are less effective than PPIs for long-term maintenance therapy or prevention of esophagitis recurrence.

5. **Adverse Effects:**

H2RAs are generally well-tolerated, with few adverse effects reported.

Rare adverse effects may include headache, dizziness, gastrointestinal disturbances, and, in the case of cimetidine, drug interactions due to its inhibition of cytochrome P450 enzymes.

Combination Therapy and Step-Up Approach:

1. **Combination Therapy:**

In refractory cases or severe esophagitis, combination therapy with PPIs and H2RAs may be considered to achieve greater acid suppression and enhance mucosal healing.

The addition of H2RAs may provide synergistic effects by targeting different steps in the gastric acid secretion pathway.

2. **Step-Up Approach:**

A step-up treatment approach involves starting with less potent acid-suppressive therapy (e.g., H2RAs) and escalating to PPIs if symptom control or mucosal healing is inadequate.

This approach may be suitable for mild cases of esophagitis or patients with minimal symptoms who may not require immediate initiation of PPI therapy.

In summary, acid-suppressive therapy with PPIs and H2RAs plays a central role in the management of esophagitis, offering effective symptom relief, mucosal healing, and prevention of disease recurrence. PPIs are preferred for moderate to severe esophagitis due to their superior efficacy and healing rates, while H2RAs may be considered for mild cases or as adjunctive therapy in refractory cases. Individualized treatment strategies, including combination therapy and step-up approaches, should be tailored to the severity of esophagitis, patient preferences, and response to initial therapy. Close monitoring and regular follow-up are essential to assess treatment response, optimize acid suppression, and minimize potential adverse effects.

Mucosal Protectants and Cytoprotective Agents

In addition to acid-suppressive therapy, mucosal protectants and cytoprotective agents play an important role in the management of esophagitis by promoting mucosal healing, enhancing barrier function, and reducing tissue inflammation. These agents provide additional therapeutic benefits, particularly in cases of erosive or ulcerative esophagitis where mucosal injury is prominent.

Sucralfate:

1. Mechanism of Action:

Sucralfate is an aluminum salt of sucrose sulfate that forms a viscous gel-like substance when exposed to gastric acid.

It adheres to ulcerated or inflamed mucosa, forming a protective barrier that shields the underlying tissue from further injury.

Additionally, sucralfate may stimulate local prostaglandin and growth factor release, promoting mucosal regeneration and repair.

2. Efficacy in Esophagitis:

Sucralfate has been shown to accelerate healing of mucosal erosions and ulcers in erosive esophagitis, providing symptomatic relief and reducing the severity of reflux symptoms.

Its cytoprotective properties make it particularly beneficial in cases of NSAID-induced esophagitis or stress-related mucosal injury.

3. Dosage and Administration:

Sucralfate is administered orally, typically as a suspension or tablet formulation.

It is recommended to be taken on an empty stomach, preferably 1 hour before meals and at bedtime, to maximize contact time with the esophageal mucosa.

4. Adverse Effects:

Sucralfate is generally well-tolerated, with minimal systemic absorption and few adverse effects reported.

Constipation, nausea, and aluminum accumulation in patients with renal impairment are potential side effects, although rare.

Alginate Formulations:

1. Mechanism of Action:

Alginate-based formulations, such as alginate-antacid combinations, work by forming a raft-like barrier on the surface of gastric contents, preventing reflux into the esophagus.

Alginate rafts create a physical barrier that floats on top of gastric contents, reducing acid contact time with the esophageal mucosa and providing symptomatic relief from heartburn and regurgitation.

2. **Efficacy in Esophagitis:**

Alginate-antacid formulations are effective in providing rapid relief from reflux symptoms, including heartburn and regurgitation, by forming a protective barrier in the esophagus. While primarily used for symptom relief rather than mucosal healing, alginate formulations may complement acid-suppressive therapy in managing mild to moderate esophagitis.

3. **Dosage and Administration:**

Alginate-antacid formulations are available as chewable tablets or liquid suspensions for oral administration.

They are typically taken as needed for symptom relief, either after meals or at bedtime, or as directed by a healthcare provider.

4. **Adverse Effects:**

Alginate formulations are generally well-tolerated, with few adverse effects reported.

Rare side effects may include gastrointestinal disturbances such as bloating, flatulence, or diarrhea.

Other Cytoprotective Agents:

1. **Misoprostol:**

Misoprostol is a synthetic prostaglandin E1 analog that promotes mucosal protection by increasing mucus production, enhancing mucosal blood flow, and inhibiting gastric acid secretion.

While primarily used for preventing NSAID-induced gastropathy, misoprostol may have a role in managing NSAID-induced esophagitis in select cases.

2. **Bismuth Compounds:**

Bismuth compounds, such as bismuth subsalicylate or bismuth

subcitrate, exert cytoprotective effects by forming a protective coating on the gastrointestinal mucosa.

While less commonly used for esophagitis, bismuth compounds may provide symptomatic relief from reflux symptoms and promote mucosal healing in erosive disease.

In summary, mucosal protectants and cytoprotective agents offer additional therapeutic benefits in the management of esophagitis by promoting mucosal healing, enhancing barrier function, and reducing tissue inflammation. Sucralfate, alginate formulations, and other cytoprotective agents may be used alone or in combination with acid-suppressive therapy to alleviate symptoms, accelerate mucosal repair, and improve patient outcomes. Individualized treatment strategies should be tailored to the severity of esophagitis, underlying etiology, and patient preferences, with close monitoring to assess treatment response and optimize therapeutic outcomes.

Topical Steroids and Anti-inflammatory Agents

In the management of esophagitis, particularly in cases of eosinophilic esophagitis (EoE) or other inflammatory conditions, topical steroids and anti-inflammatory agents play a crucial role in reducing esophageal inflammation, suppressing immune-mediated responses, and promoting mucosal healing. These agents target underlying inflammatory processes, providing symptomatic relief and preventing disease progression.

Topical Steroids:

1. **Mechanism of Action:**

Topical corticosteroids exert anti-inflammatory effects by inhibiting the synthesis of pro-inflammatory cytokines, suppressing immune cell activation, and reducing tissue inflammation.

When administered topically to the esophagus, corticosteroids target local inflammatory processes, attenuating eosinophilic infiltration and mucosal inflammation.

2. **Efficacy in Esophagitis:**

Topical steroids are highly effective in inducing remission and maintaining disease control in eosinophilic esophagitis, the most common cause of non-reflux esophagitis.

They reduce esophageal eosinophilia, improve symptoms such as dysphagia and food impaction, and promote mucosal healing, as demonstrated in clinical trials and observational studies.

3. **Types of Topical Steroids:**

Swallowed Steroids: Budesonide oral suspension or fluticasone propionate inhalers are commonly used as swallowed formulations for topical delivery to the esophagus.

Topical Sprays: Steroid sprays or aerosols, such as ciclesonide or fluticasone, may be directly sprayed onto the esophageal mucosa during endoscopic procedures for localized delivery.

4. **Dosage and Administration:**

Swallowed Steroids: Budesonide oral suspension is typically administered orally, either as a single daily dose or divided doses, with instructions to hold the medication in the mouth before swallowing.

Topical Sprays: Steroid sprays are administered directly onto the esophageal mucosa during endoscopy, with subsequent swallowing to distribute the medication throughout the esophagus.

5. **Adverse Effects:**

Topical steroids are generally safe and well-tolerated when used appropriately for short-term or intermittent courses.

Potential adverse effects include local irritation, dysphagia, or candidiasis, particularly with prolonged or high-dose therapy.

Anti-inflammatory Agents:

1. **5-Aminosalicylates (5-ASA):**

5-ASA agents, such as mesalamine or balsalazide, have anti-inflammatory properties and may be beneficial in certain cases of esophagitis, including eosinophilic esophagitis or reflux esophagitis with concomitant inflammatory bowel disease (IBD).

Oral or rectal formulations of 5-ASA may be considered for patients with concurrent esophageal and gastrointestinal inflammation.

2. **Immunomodulators:**

Immunomodulatory agents, such as azathioprine, 6-mercaptopurine, or methotrexate, may be used as adjunctive therapy in refractory cases of eosinophilic esophagitis or autoimmune esophagitis.

These agents modulate immune responses, suppress T-cell activation, and reduce cytokine production, thereby attenuating esophageal inflammation.

3. **Biologic Therapies:**

Biologic agents targeting specific inflammatory pathways, such as interleukin-5 (IL-5) inhibitors (e.g., mepolizumab, reslizumab) or anti-interleukin-13 (IL-13) antibodies (e.g., dupilumab), have shown promise in the treatment of eosinophilic esophagitis.

Biologics selectively block key mediators of eosinophilic inflammation, reducing eosinophil counts, improving symptoms, and promoting mucosal healing.

In summary, topical steroids and anti-inflammatory agents play a crucial role in the management of esophagitis, particularly in cases of eosinophilic esophagitis or other inflammatory conditions. These agents target underlying inflammation, reduce esophageal eosinophilia, alleviate symptoms, and promote mucosal healing. Individualized treatment approaches, incorporating topical corticosteroids, anti-inflammatory agents, and immunomodulatory therapies, should be tailored to the underlying etiology, disease severity, and patient preferences, with close monitoring to assess treatment response and optimize therapeutic outcomes.

Role of Immunomodulatory Drugs and Biologics

In the management of esophagitis, particularly in cases of refractory or autoimmune-mediated disease, immunomodulatory drugs and biologic agents play a pivotal role in modulating immune responses, reducing inflammation, and promoting mucosal healing. These advanced therapies target specific pathways involved in esophageal inflammation, offering new treatment options for patients with challenging or severe forms of esophagitis.

Immunomodulatory Drugs:

1. **Azathioprine and 6-Mercaptopurine:**

Azathioprine and its metabolite, 6-mercaptopurine, are thiopurine analogs that inhibit purine synthesis and suppress T-cell proliferation.

These agents are used as steroid-sparing therapies in refractory cases of eosinophilic esophagitis, autoimmune esophagitis, or Crohn's disease-associated esophagitis.

2. **Methotrexate:**

Methotrexate is a folate antagonist that interferes with DNA synthesis and cell proliferation, exerting immunosuppressive effects.

It may be used as an alternative or adjunctive therapy in refractory cases of autoimmune esophagitis or eosinophilic esophagitis, particularly in patients intolerant of or unresponsive to other immunomodulatory agents.

Biologic Therapies:

1. Interleukin-5 (IL-5) Inhibitors:

IL-5 inhibitors, such as mepolizumab and reslizumab, target eosinophilic inflammation by blocking the action of IL-5, a key cytokine involved in eosinophil activation and recruitment.

These biologics reduce esophageal eosinophilia, improve symptoms, and promote mucosal healing in patients with eosinophilic esophagitis who are refractory to standard therapies.

2. Anti-Interleukin-13 (IL-13) Antibodies:

Anti-IL-13 antibodies, such as dupilumab, inhibit the signaling of IL-13, a cytokine implicated in the pathogenesis of eosinophilic esophagitis and other Th2-mediated inflammatory disorders.

Dupilumab has shown efficacy in reducing esophageal eosinophilia, improving symptoms, and achieving histologic remission in patients with moderate to severe eosinophilic esophagitis.

3. Tumor Necrosis Factor-alpha (TNF-α) Inhibitors:

TNF-α inhibitors, including infliximab, adalimumab, and certolizumab, block the action of TNF-α, a pro-inflammatory cytokine involved in the pathogenesis of autoimmune and inflammatory conditions.

While not specifically approved for esophagitis, TNF-α inhibitors may be considered in refractory cases of autoimmune esophagitis or Crohn's disease-associated esophagitis.

4. Other Biologic Agents:

Emerging biologic therapies targeting novel pathways involved in esophageal inflammation are currently under investigation for the treatment of esophagitis.

These include anti-IL-4/IL-13 antibodies, anti-Siglec-8 antibodies, and other agents targeting specific immune cell populations or cytokine signaling pathways.

Patient Selection and Monitoring:

1. **Patient Selection:**

Selection of immunomodulatory drugs and biologic therapies should be based on the underlying etiology, disease severity, treatment goals, and individual patient factors.

Referral to gastroenterologists or immunologists with expertise in esophageal disorders is recommended for appropriate patient evaluation and treatment decision-making.

2. **Monitoring and Adverse Effects:**

Regular monitoring of patients receiving immunomodulatory drugs or biologic therapies is essential to assess treatment response, monitor for adverse effects, and optimize therapeutic outcomes.

Adverse effects may include immunosuppression, increased risk of infections, infusion reactions, or other medication-specific side effects, necessitating close supervision and proactive management.

In summary, immunomodulatory drugs and biologic therapies represent promising treatment options for refractory or autoimmune-mediated esophagitis, offering targeted modulation of immune responses and inflammation. These advanced therapies have demonstrated efficacy in reducing esophageal inflammation, improving symptoms, and promoting mucosal healing in select patient populations. Individualized treatment approaches, guided by disease-specific considerations and patient preferences, should be tailored to optimize therapeutic outcomes and enhance quality of life for individuals with challenging forms of esophagitis. Close collaboration between gastroenterologists, allergists, and immunologists is essential for comprehensive patient care and management of esophageal disorders.

CHAPTER 11: NON-PHARMACOLOGICAL INTERVENTIONS AND LIFESTYLE MODIFICATIONS

Dietary Modifications and Nutritional Considerations

Dietary modifications and nutritional interventions play a crucial role in the management of esophagitis, aiming to reduce symptoms, minimize esophageal irritation, promote mucosal healing, and improve overall health and well-being. Various dietary strategies, including avoidance of trigger foods, modification of meal timing and composition, and optimization of nutritional intake, are employed to alleviate symptoms and support optimal esophageal health.

Identifying Trigger Foods:

1. **Acidic Foods and Beverages:**
Citrus fruits, tomatoes, and acidic juices (e.g., orange juice, grapefruit juice) can exacerbate reflux symptoms and

esophageal irritation due to their high acidity.
Carbonated beverages, caffeinated drinks (e.g., coffee, tea), and alcoholic beverages may also trigger reflux and worsen esophagitis symptoms.

2. Spicy and Irritating Foods:

Spicy foods, peppermint, chocolate, and high-fat meals are known to relax the lower esophageal sphincter (LES) and increase the risk of acid reflux and heartburn.
Foods with rough or coarse textures, such as dry crackers or chips, may irritate the esophageal mucosa and exacerbate symptoms.

3. High-Fat and Fried Foods:

High-fat foods, fried foods, and greasy or heavy meals can delay gastric emptying, increase gastric acid production, and promote reflux into the esophagus.
Opting for lower-fat cooking methods (e.g., grilling, steaming) and choosing lean protein sources may help reduce symptoms of reflux and esophagitis.

Meal Timing and Composition:

1. Small, Frequent Meals:

Consuming smaller, more frequent meals throughout the day can help prevent excessive gastric distention and reduce pressure on the LES, minimizing reflux episodes.
Snacking on light, easily digestible foods between meals may help maintain satiety and prevent overeating.

2. Early Dinner and Bedtime Snacks:

Avoiding heavy or large meals within 2-3 hours of bedtime can reduce the risk of nocturnal reflux and promote better sleep quality.
Bedtime snacks should be light and reflux-friendly, such as non-acidic fruits (e.g., bananas, apples), whole-grain crackers, or low-fat dairy products.

3. Meal Composition:

Emphasizing a plant-based diet rich in fruits, vegetables, whole grains, and legumes can provide essential nutrients, fiber, and antioxidants while reducing the intake of potential trigger foods.

Including lean protein sources (e.g., poultry, fish, tofu) and healthy fats (e.g., avocados, nuts, olive oil) in meals can help promote satiety and support balanced nutrition.

Nutritional Considerations:

1. **Maintaining Adequate Hydration:**

Adequate hydration is essential for maintaining optimal esophageal health, promoting mucosal hydration, and facilitating swallowing.

Drinking plenty of water throughout the day, particularly between meals, can help soothe the esophagus and prevent symptoms of dryness or irritation.

2. **Optimizing Fiber Intake:**

Dietary fiber plays a crucial role in promoting gastrointestinal motility, preventing constipation, and reducing the risk of esophageal reflux.

Consuming fiber-rich foods such as whole grains, fruits, vegetables, and legumes can help regulate bowel movements and alleviate symptoms of gastroesophageal reflux disease (GERD).

3. **Supplementing with Vitamins and Minerals:**

Certain vitamins and minerals, such as vitamin C, vitamin E, and zinc, have antioxidant properties that may help protect the esophageal mucosa from oxidative stress and inflammation.

Incorporating a balanced diet with a variety of nutrient-rich foods can help ensure adequate intake of essential vitamins and minerals necessary for optimal esophageal health.

Individualized Approach and Dietary Counseling:

1. **Tailoring Dietary Recommendations:**

Dietary modifications should be individualized based on the patient's specific triggers, symptom severity, nutritional needs, and personal preferences.

Working closely with a registered dietitian or nutritionist can help develop personalized meal plans, identify trigger foods, and address nutritional deficiencies while promoting overall health and well-being.

2. **Monitoring and Adjusting:**

Regular monitoring of dietary intake, symptom response, and nutritional status is essential for evaluating the effectiveness of dietary modifications and making appropriate adjustments as needed.

Keeping a food diary or symptom journal can help patients identify patterns, track triggers, and make informed decisions about dietary choices.

In summary, dietary modifications and nutritional considerations are integral components of the management of esophagitis, offering a holistic approach to symptom management and mucosal healing. By identifying trigger foods, optimizing meal timing and composition, and addressing nutritional needs, patients can alleviate symptoms, minimize esophageal irritation, and support overall esophageal health. Individualized dietary counseling and ongoing monitoring play a crucial role in achieving optimal outcomes and improving quality of life for individuals with esophagitis.

Behavioral Strategies: Weight Management and Positional Therapy

Behavioral strategies, including weight management and positional therapy, are integral components of the holistic management of esophagitis. These approaches focus on modifying lifestyle habits and behaviors to reduce symptoms, minimize esophageal irritation, and optimize esophageal health.

Weight Management:

1. Impact of Obesity on Esophagitis:

Obesity is a significant risk factor for the development and exacerbation of esophagitis, particularly gastroesophageal reflux disease (GERD) and erosive esophagitis.

Excess abdominal fat can increase intra-abdominal pressure, leading to transient relaxation of the lower esophageal sphincter (LES) and promoting reflux of gastric contents into the esophagus.

2. Benefits of Weight Loss:

Weight loss can improve symptoms of GERD and esophagitis by reducing intra-abdominal pressure, enhancing LES function, and decreasing the frequency and severity of reflux episodes.

Even modest weight reduction (e.g., 5-10% of total body weight) has been shown to result in significant improvements in GERD symptoms and esophageal inflammation.

3. Strategies for Weight Management:

Adopting a balanced, calorie-controlled diet rich in fruits, vegetables, whole grains, and lean protein sources can support weight loss and promote overall health.

Incorporating regular physical activity, such as aerobic exercise and strength training, can help burn calories, improve metabolism, and facilitate weight loss.

Positional Therapy:

1. Impact of Body Position on Reflux:

Body positioning, particularly during sleep, can influence the occurrence and severity of nocturnal reflux episodes in patients with esophagitis.

Sleeping in a supine (flat) position allows gastric contents to more easily reflux into the esophagus, exacerbating symptoms and increasing the risk of esophageal irritation.

   2. **Benefits of Elevated Sleeping Position:**

Elevating the head of the bed or using a wedge pillow to raise the upper body during sleep can reduce the frequency and duration of reflux episodes by gravity-assisted clearance of gastric contents.

Sleeping in a semi-upright position helps prevent acid from pooling in the esophagus, minimizing contact time with the esophageal mucosa and reducing the risk of mucosal injury.

   3. **Positional Therapy Devices:**

Wedge pillows, bed risers, or adjustable bed frames can be used to elevate the head of the bed, creating a slight incline that promotes drainage of gastric contents away from the esophagus. Alternatively, positional therapy devices, such as wearable devices or sleep positioning belts, can help maintain a side-sleeping position, which may be associated with reduced reflux compared to sleeping in a supine position.

Combination of Behavioral Strategies:

   1. **Synergistic Effects:**

Combining weight management with positional therapy can synergistically reduce the severity and frequency of reflux episodes, providing comprehensive symptom relief and improving esophageal health.

Weight loss reduces intra-abdominal pressure and LES dysfunction, while positional therapy minimizes nocturnal reflux and esophageal exposure to gastric acid.

   2. **Patient Education and Adherence:**

Patient education is essential for promoting adherence to behavioral strategies and fostering long-term lifestyle modifications.

Providing information on the benefits of weight management, proper positioning during sleep, and practical tips for incorporating these strategies into daily routines can empower patients to take an active role in managing their esophagitis.

In summary, behavioral strategies, including weight management and positional therapy, play a vital role in the holistic management of esophagitis, complementing pharmacological and dietary interventions. By promoting weight loss, adopting proper body positioning during sleep, and integrating these strategies into daily routines, patients can effectively reduce reflux symptoms, minimize esophageal irritation, and improve overall esophageal health. Individualized counseling, patient education, and ongoing support are essential for encouraging adherence to behavioral modifications and optimizing therapeutic outcomes for individuals with esophagitis.

Avoidance of Triggering Factors: Smoking, Alcohol, and Caffeine

In the management of esophagitis, avoiding triggering factors such as smoking, alcohol, and caffeine is crucial for minimizing symptoms, reducing esophageal irritation, and promoting overall esophageal health. These lifestyle habits can exacerbate reflux symptoms, increase esophageal inflammation, and contribute to the development or progression of esophagitis.

Smoking:

1. **Impact on Esophageal Health:**
Smoking is a well-established risk factor for gastroesophageal reflux disease (GERD) and erosive esophagitis due to its effects on lower esophageal sphincter (LES) function and esophageal motility.
Nicotine in tobacco smoke can relax the LES, impair esophageal clearance, and increase acid reflux into the esophagus, leading to

mucosal injury and inflammation.

2. **Benefits of Smoking Cessation:**

Quitting smoking has been shown to significantly reduce the severity and frequency of reflux symptoms, improve LES function, and decrease the risk of esophagitis and its complications.

Smokers who quit experience rapid improvements in esophageal health, with reductions in reflux episodes and resolution of esophageal inflammation over time.

Alcohol:

1. **Effect on Esophageal Function:**

Alcohol consumption is associated with an increased risk of GERD, erosive esophagitis, and Barrett's esophagus, primarily through its effects on LES tone and esophageal motility.

- Alcohol can relax the LES, delay gastric emptying, and promote reflux of acidic gastric contents into the esophagus, exacerbating symptoms and causing esophageal injury.

2. **Moderation and Avoidance:**

Limiting or avoiding alcohol consumption, particularly before bedtime or in large quantities, can help reduce the risk of reflux and minimize esophageal irritation.

Moderate alcohol consumption, defined as up to one drink per day for women and up to two drinks per day for men, may be acceptable for some individuals without exacerbating reflux symptoms.

Caffeine:

1. **Impact on Acid Reflux:**

Caffeine, found in coffee, tea, energy drinks, and certain medications, can stimulate gastric acid secretion and relax the LES, contributing to reflux episodes and worsening esophagitis symptoms.

High caffeine intake, especially in the form of strong coffee or caffeinated beverages, has been linked to an increased risk of GERD and erosive esophagitis.

2. **Reducing Caffeine Consumption:**

Limiting caffeine intake, particularly in the evening or before bedtime, can help reduce nighttime reflux and improve sleep quality.

Choosing decaffeinated options or caffeine-free beverages may be preferable for individuals sensitive to caffeine or prone to reflux symptoms.

Integrated Approach:

1. **Patient Education and Behavior Modification:**

Patient education plays a central role in promoting awareness of the detrimental effects of smoking, alcohol, and caffeine on esophageal health.

Encouraging behavior modification strategies, such as smoking cessation programs, alcohol moderation, and caffeine reduction, can empower individuals to make positive lifestyle changes and improve their esophageal symptoms.

2. **Supportive Resources and Counseling:**

Providing access to supportive resources, such as smoking cessation programs, alcohol counseling services, and dietary counseling, can facilitate behavior change and enhance adherence to lifestyle modifications.

Offering personalized counseling and ongoing support can address individual challenges, barriers to change, and concerns related to lifestyle modifications.

In summary, avoidance of triggering factors such as smoking, alcohol, and caffeine is essential for the management of esophagitis, as these lifestyle habits can exacerbate reflux symptoms and contribute to esophageal inflammation. By quitting smoking, moderating alcohol consumption, and reducing caffeine intake, individuals can minimize esophageal irritation, improve LES function, and promote overall esophageal health. Integrated strategies that combine patient education, behavior modification, and supportive resources are key to facilitating long-term adherence to lifestyle modifications and optimizing therapeutic outcomes for individuals with esophagitis.

Stress Reduction Techniques and Psychological Support

In the management of esophagitis, stress reduction techniques and psychological support play a crucial role in alleviating symptoms, reducing esophageal inflammation, and improving overall quality of life. Psychological factors, including stress, anxiety, and depression, can exacerbate reflux symptoms and contribute to esophageal hypersensitivity, highlighting the importance of addressing both physical and emotional aspects of esophageal health.

Impact of Stress on Esophagitis:

1. **Stress-Induced Symptoms:**

Stress and emotional distress can exacerbate symptoms of gastroesophageal reflux disease (GERD) and esophagitis by increasing gastric acid secretion, altering esophageal motility, and enhancing visceral sensitivity.

Chronic stress may exacerbate inflammation and impair mucosal healing in the esophagus, leading to persistent or recurrent symptoms despite medical therapy.

2. **Psychological Comorbidities:**

Individuals with esophagitis are more likely to experience psychological comorbidities, such as anxiety, depression, or somatization disorders, which can contribute to symptom severity and treatment resistance.

Psychological distress can also impact adherence to dietary and lifestyle modifications, pharmacological therapies, and follow-up care, further complicating the management of esophageal disorders.

Stress Reduction Techniques:

1. Mindfulness and Relaxation Techniques:

Mindfulness-based stress reduction (MBSR), meditation, deep breathing exercises, and progressive muscle relaxation techniques can help reduce sympathetic nervous system activity, promote relaxation, and alleviate stress-related symptoms.

Practicing mindfulness and relaxation techniques regularly can improve coping mechanisms, enhance emotional resilience, and reduce the impact of stress on esophageal symptoms.

2. Cognitive-Behavioral Therapy (CBT):

CBT is a structured psychotherapeutic approach that helps individuals identify and modify maladaptive thought patterns, behaviors, and coping strategies related to stress and anxiety.

CBT techniques, including cognitive restructuring, relaxation training, and stress management skills, have been shown to be effective in reducing reflux symptoms and improving quality of life in patients with GERD and esophagitis.

3. Yoga and Exercise:

Yoga, tai chi, and other mind-body exercises combine physical activity with mindfulness and relaxation techniques, offering holistic benefits for both physical and emotional well-being.

Regular exercise, such as walking, swimming, or cycling, can help reduce stress, improve mood, and enhance overall health, contributing to better management of esophageal symptoms.

Psychological Support:

1. Individual Counseling and Support Groups:

Individual counseling with a psychologist or mental health professional can provide personalized support, coping strategies, and psychoeducation tailored to the unique needs of individuals with esophagitis.

Participating in support groups or online forums can offer peer support, validation, and encouragement from others with similar experiences, fostering a sense of community and belonging.

2. **Integrated Care Approach:**

Collaborative care models that integrate psychological support into the management of esophagitis, such as multidisciplinary clinics or gastroenterology-psychiatry partnerships, can address both physical and emotional aspects of the condition.

Coordinated efforts between gastroenterologists, psychologists, dietitians, and other healthcare providers can optimize treatment outcomes, enhance patient satisfaction, and improve overall quality of life for individuals with esophagitis.

Patient Education and Empowerment:

1. **Promoting Self-Care and Resilience:**

Patient education plays a vital role in promoting self-care strategies, stress management techniques, and resilience-building skills to empower individuals to take an active role in managing their esophageal symptoms.

Providing information on the impact of stress on esophageal health, coping mechanisms for stress reduction, and available resources for psychological support can empower patients to make informed decisions and advocate for their well-being.

2. **Addressing Stigma and Misconceptions:**

Addressing stigma, shame, and misconceptions surrounding mental health and gastrointestinal disorders can help reduce barriers to seeking psychological support and improve access to integrated care.

Educating patients, families, and healthcare providers about the bidirectional relationship between stress and esophageal health can foster empathy, understanding, and collaborative decision-making in the management of esophagitis.

In summary, stress reduction techniques and psychological support are essential components of the holistic management of esophagitis, addressing the interplay between emotional well-being and esophageal health. By incorporating mindfulness, relaxation techniques, cognitive-behavioral interventions, and psychological support into comprehensive care plans, healthcare providers can help individuals with esophagitis better cope with stress, reduce symptom severity, and improve overall quality of life. Integrated approaches that combine physical, dietary, and psychological interventions can optimize treatment outcomes and promote long-term well-being for individuals living with esophagitis.

CHAPTER 12: INTEGRATIVE AND HOLISTIC APPROACHES TO ESOPHAGITIS MANAGEMENT

Herbal and Nutraceutical Therapies

In addition to conventional pharmacological treatments, herbal and nutraceutical therapies offer alternative or complementary approaches to managing esophagitis. Derived from natural sources, including plants, herbs, and dietary supplements, these interventions aim to alleviate symptoms, reduce esophageal inflammation, and promote mucosal healing. While scientific evidence supporting their efficacy is often limited, certain herbal remedies and nutraceuticals have shown promise in preclinical studies and clinical trials for the management of esophageal disorders.

Herbal Therapies:

1. **Aloe Vera:**

Aloe vera has anti-inflammatory and mucoprotective properties, making it a popular remedy for gastrointestinal conditions, including esophagitis.

Oral supplementation with aloe vera juice or gel may help soothe esophageal irritation, reduce inflammation, and promote healing of the esophageal mucosa.

2. **Marshmallow Root (Althaea officinalis):**

Marshmallow root contains mucilaginous compounds that form a protective layer over the esophageal mucosa, reducing irritation and enhancing mucosal barrier function.

Herbal teas or extracts of marshmallow root may be used to alleviate symptoms of esophagitis, such as heartburn, dysphagia, and throat discomfort.

3. **Licorice (Glycyrrhiza glabra):**

Licorice root contains glycyrrhizin, a compound with anti-inflammatory and mucoprotective effects that may help reduce esophageal inflammation and promote healing.

Deglycyrrhizinated licorice (DGL) supplements, which have had the glycyrrhizin removed to prevent side effects, are commonly used for the management of GERD and erosive esophagitis.

4. **Chamomile (Matricaria chamomilla):**

Chamomile is known for its calming and anti-inflammatory properties, which may help alleviate symptoms of esophagitis, such as reflux and dyspepsia.

Chamomile tea or supplements may be used as a natural remedy to soothe esophageal irritation and reduce inflammation.

Nutraceutical Therapies:

1. **Deglycyrrhizinated Licorice (DGL):**

DGL supplements have been studied for their potential to increase mucosal resistance, enhance mucin secretion, and reduce gastric acid secretion, making them a popular adjunctive therapy for GERD and esophagitis.

DGL may help protect the esophageal mucosa from damage caused by acid reflux and promote healing of erosive lesions.

2. **Melatonin:**

Melatonin, a hormone produced by the pineal gland, has antioxidant, anti-inflammatory, and gastroprotective effects that may benefit individuals with esophagitis.

Melatonin supplementation has been shown to improve symptoms of GERD, reduce esophageal inflammation, and enhance esophageal motility in clinical studies.

3. **Omega-3 Fatty Acids:**

Omega-3 fatty acids, found in fish oil and certain plant-based sources, possess anti-inflammatory properties that may help reduce esophageal inflammation and promote healing.

Supplementation with omega-3 fatty acids has been investigated as a potential adjunctive therapy for inflammatory conditions of the esophagus, including eosinophilic esophagitis.

4. **Probiotics:**

Probiotics are live microorganisms that confer health benefits when consumed in adequate amounts, including modulation of the gut microbiota and modulation of immune responses.

Certain probiotic strains, such as Lactobacillus and Bifidobacterium species, may help maintain gut health, reduce inflammation, and improve symptoms in individuals with esophagitis.

Safety and Considerations:

1. **Quality and Standardization:**

Quality control and standardization of herbal and nutraceutical products are essential to ensure purity, potency, and consistency of active ingredients.

Choosing reputable brands with third-party certification (e.g., USP, NSF) can help minimize the risk of contamination and ensure product efficacy.

2. **Potential Interactions:**

Herbal and nutraceutical therapies may interact with medications or other supplements, potentially affecting their efficacy or safety.

Patients should consult with healthcare providers before initiating herbal or nutraceutical therapies, especially if they are taking prescription medications or have underlying medical conditions.

3. **Individualized Approach:**

Herbal and nutraceutical therapies should be individualized based on the underlying etiology, symptom severity, and patient preferences.

Integrative healthcare providers, including naturopathic physicians or integrative medicine specialists, can help guide treatment decisions and monitor patient response to herbal and nutraceutical interventions.

In summary, herbal and nutraceutical therapies offer alternative or adjunctive approaches to managing esophagitis, providing natural remedies with potential benefits for symptom relief and mucosal healing. While scientific evidence supporting their efficacy is evolving, certain herbal remedies and nutraceuticals have shown promise in preclinical and clinical studies for the management of esophageal disorders. Patient education, safety considerations, and individualized treatment approaches are essential for optimizing the use of herbal and nutraceutical therapies in the management of esophagitis.

Acupuncture and Traditional Chinese Medicine

Acupuncture and Traditional Chinese Medicine (TCM) offer holistic approaches to the management of esophagitis, focusing on restoring balance and harmony within the body to alleviate symptoms, reduce inflammation, and promote overall well-being. Rooted in ancient principles and techniques, acupuncture and TCM modalities aim to address underlying imbalances in the body's energy flow, known as Qi, and restore health through the stimulation of specific points along meridians.

Acupuncture:

1. Principles and Mechanisms:

Acupuncture involves the insertion of thin needles into specific acupuncture points along meridians, aiming to regulate the flow of Qi and restore balance within the body.

By stimulating acupuncture points related to the digestive system, such as those along the Stomach and Spleen meridians, acupuncture may help regulate gastrointestinal function, reduce inflammation, and alleviate symptoms of esophagitis.

2. Clinical Evidence and Efficacy:

Clinical studies evaluating the efficacy of acupuncture for gastroesophageal reflux disease (GERD) and esophagitis have shown promising results, with some demonstrating improvements in reflux symptoms, esophageal inflammation, and quality of life.

Acupuncture may modulate esophageal sphincter function, enhance esophageal motility, and reduce acid reflux by regulating neural pathways, neurotransmitter levels, and autonomic nervous system activity.

Traditional Chinese Herbal Medicine:

1. Herbal Formulations and Prescriptions:

Traditional Chinese Herbal Medicine (TCM) utilizes a variety of herbal formulations and prescriptions tailored to individual patterns of disharmony, known as syndromes, based on TCM diagnostic principles.

Herbal remedies for esophagitis may include combinations of

herbs with anti-inflammatory, mucoprotective, and digestive properties, aiming to address underlying imbalances and alleviate symptoms.

2. **Clinical Applications and Evidence:**

Clinical studies investigating the efficacy of TCM herbal formulations for GERD and esophagitis have shown mixed results, with some demonstrating symptom improvement and reduction in esophageal inflammation.

TCM herbal medicine may target various aspects of esophageal dysfunction, including excessive acid secretion, impaired motility, and mucosal injury, through multifaceted mechanisms of action.

Dietary Therapy and Lifestyle Recommendations:

1. **Dietary Modifications:**

TCM dietary therapy emphasizes the importance of balancing flavors, temperatures, and energetic properties of foods to support digestive health and promote harmony within the body. Recommendations may include avoiding spicy, greasy, or irritating foods, consuming smaller, more frequent meals, and incorporating foods with cooling or nourishing properties to soothe esophageal inflammation.

2. **Lifestyle Recommendations:**

TCM emphasizes the interconnectedness of physical, emotional, and environmental factors in health and disease, recommending lifestyle modifications to reduce stress, enhance relaxation, and support overall well-being.

Techniques such as qigong, tai chi, and meditation may be recommended to promote relaxation, reduce stress, and cultivate mindfulness, complementing acupuncture and herbal interventions for esophagitis.

Integration with Conventional Care:

1. **Collaborative Approach:**

Integrating acupuncture and TCM with conventional medical care for esophagitis allows for a comprehensive, patient-centered approach that addresses both the symptoms and underlying imbalances contributing to the condition.

Collaborative efforts between TCM practitioners, gastroenterologists, and other healthcare providers can optimize treatment outcomes, improve symptom management, and enhance overall quality of life for individuals with esophagitis.

2. **Individualized Treatment Plans:**

TCM recognizes the unique constitution, patterns of disharmony, and treatment responses of each individual, tailoring treatment plans and herbal prescriptions to address specific needs and preferences.

Patient education, empowerment, and active participation in treatment decisions are emphasized, fostering a sense of partnership and collaboration in the healing process.

In summary, acupuncture and Traditional Chinese Medicine offer holistic approaches to the management of esophagitis, addressing both the symptoms and underlying imbalances contributing to the condition. By restoring balance within the body, regulating Qi flow, and promoting overall well-being, these modalities complement conventional medical therapies and provide additional options for individuals seeking alternative or integrative approaches to esophageal health. Individualized treatment plans, collaborative care, and ongoing support are essential for optimizing outcomes and promoting long-term wellness for individuals with esophagitis.

CHAPTER 13: SURGICAL MANAGEMENT OF ESOPHAGITIS AND REFRACTORY CASES

Indications for Surgical Intervention

Surgical intervention for esophagitis is typically reserved for cases where conservative medical management fails to adequately control symptoms or when complications such as strictures, Barrett's esophagus, or severe erosive disease develop. Surgical options aim to address the underlying anatomical abnormalities contributing to reflux and esophageal injury, thereby providing long-term relief and preventing disease progression. Indications for surgical intervention in esophagitis include:

1. **Failure of Medical Therapy:**
Persistent symptoms despite optimal medical management

with proton pump inhibitors (PPIs), histamine-2 receptor antagonists (H2RAs), or other acid-suppressive medications may indicate the need for surgical intervention.

Individuals who experience incomplete symptom relief, breakthrough symptoms, or recurrent erosive esophagitis despite adherence to medical therapy may benefit from surgical correction of underlying anatomical defects.

2. **Complications of Reflux Disease:**

Complications such as esophageal strictures, Barrett's esophagus, or recurrent esophageal ulcers may necessitate surgical intervention to prevent disease progression and reduce the risk of long-term complications.

Surgical correction of anatomical abnormalities, such as hiatal hernia repair or fundoplication, can help prevent reflux-induced damage to the esophagus and reduce the risk of complications associated with chronic reflux disease.

3. **Refractory Esophagitis:**

Refractory esophagitis, characterized by persistent or recurrent inflammation and mucosal injury despite aggressive medical therapy, may require surgical intervention to address underlying anatomical defects and provide long-term symptom relief.

Individuals with severe erosive esophagitis, esophageal ulcers, or complications such as esophageal strictures that do not respond to medical treatment may benefit from surgical correction of reflux-related abnormalities.

4. **Severe Gastroesophageal Reflux Disease (GERD):**

Individuals with severe or complicated GERD, including those with severe erosive esophagitis, Barrett's esophagus with dysplasia, or extraesophageal manifestations such as asthma or laryngitis, may be candidates for surgical intervention.

Surgical options such as fundoplication or LINX (lower esophageal sphincter augmentation) may be considered in individuals with severe reflux disease who are not responsive to or intolerant of medical therapy.

5. **Younger Age and Long-Term Considerations:**

Surgical intervention may be preferred in younger individuals with esophagitis, particularly those with long life expectancies, to provide durable symptom relief and prevent complications associated with chronic reflux disease.

Long-term considerations, including the risk of medication side effects, the need for ongoing medical therapy, and the potential for disease progression, should be weighed when considering surgical options for esophagitis.

Preoperative Evaluation and Assessment:

1. **Comprehensive Clinical Evaluation:**

Prior to surgical intervention, individuals with esophagitis should undergo a comprehensive clinical evaluation, including a thorough medical history, physical examination, endoscopic evaluation, and diagnostic testing to assess the severity of reflux disease and identify any complications.

Preoperative assessment may include esophageal manometry, ambulatory pH monitoring, esophagogastroduodenoscopy (EGD), barium swallow, and imaging studies to evaluate esophageal anatomy, motility, and reflux parameters.

2. **Multidisciplinary Approach:**

The decision to pursue surgical intervention for esophagitis should be made collaboratively by a multidisciplinary team of healthcare providers, including gastroenterologists, surgeons, dietitians, and other specialists.

A comprehensive preoperative assessment ensures that individuals are well-informed about their treatment options, understand the potential risks and benefits of surgery, and are actively involved in the decision-making process.

Conclusion: Surgical intervention for esophagitis is indicated in cases of refractory symptoms, complications of reflux disease, or failure of medical therapy to adequately control symptoms. By addressing underlying anatomical abnormalities and restoring the integrity of the gastroesophageal junction, surgical options provide long-term relief and prevent disease progression in individuals with esophagitis. A comprehensive preoperative evaluation and assessment, along with a multidisciplinary approach to care, are essential for optimizing outcomes and ensuring that individuals receive appropriate surgical management tailored to their specific needs and circumstances.

Surgical Procedures: Fundoplication, Endoscopic Techniques, and Esophagectomy

Surgical intervention plays a crucial role in the management of esophagitis, offering definitive treatment options for individuals with refractory symptoms, complications of reflux disease, or failure of medical therapy. Surgical procedures aim to address underlying anatomical abnormalities, restore the integrity of the gastroesophageal junction, and provide long-term relief from reflux symptoms. Key surgical options for esophagitis include fundoplication, endoscopic techniques, and esophagectomy.

Fundoplication:

1. **Principles and Techniques:**

Fundoplication is a surgical procedure commonly used to treat gastroesophageal reflux disease (GERD) and its complications, including esophagitis and hiatal hernia.During fundoplication, the upper part of the stomach (fundus) is wrapped around the lower esophagus and secured in place to create a valve mechanism that prevents gastric reflux into the esophagus. Fundoplication may be performed via open surgery or minimally invasive techniques, such as laparoscopic or robotic-assisted surgery, depending on individual patient factors and surgeon preference.

2. **Types of Fundoplication:**

Nissen Fundoplication: The fundus of the stomach is wrapped fully around the lower esophagus, creating a 360-degree wrap, to reinforce the lower esophageal sphincter (LES) and prevent reflux.

Toupet Fundoplication: A partial 270-degree wrap of the fundus is performed around the lower esophagus, providing less tightness and potentially reducing the risk of postoperative dysphagia.

Dor Fundoplication: A partial anterior wrap is created, anchoring the anterior wall of the fundus to the anterior esophageal wall, to reinforce the LES and prevent reflux.

3. **Indications and Outcomes:**

Fundoplication is indicated for individuals with refractory symptoms of GERD, erosive esophagitis, or complications such as esophageal strictures, Barrett's esophagus, or aspiration pneumonia.

The success rate of fundoplication for GERD and esophagitis is generally high, with significant improvement or resolution of symptoms reported in the majority of patients. However, long-term outcomes may vary, and some individuals may experience recurrence of symptoms over time.

Endoscopic Techniques:

1. **Endoscopic Fundoplication (TIF):**

Transoral incisionless fundoplication (TIF) is an endoscopic procedure that aims to recreate a valve mechanism at the gastroesophageal junction to reduce reflux.

During TIF, tissue plication devices are used to create folds and tighten the junction between the esophagus and stomach, thereby improving the competence of the LES and reducing reflux.

TIF may be considered in select individuals with GERD and mild to moderate esophagitis who are not candidates for traditional surgical fundoplication or prefer less invasive treatment options.

2. **Radiofrequency Ablation (Stretta Procedure):**

The Stretta procedure is an endoscopic technique that uses radiofrequency energy to treat the lower esophageal sphincter (LES) and improve its function.

Radiofrequency energy is delivered to the LES and surrounding tissues, resulting in thermal injury and subsequent remodeling, which may lead to enhanced barrier function and reduced reflux.

Stretta may be considered in individuals with GERD and esophagitis who are not responsive to medical therapy or prefer minimally invasive treatment options.

Esophagectomy:

1. **Indications and Considerations:**

Esophagectomy is a major surgical procedure that involves the removal of part or all of the esophagus, typically in cases of advanced esophageal disease, such as severe esophagitis, Barrett's esophagus with high-grade dysplasia or carcinoma in situ, or invasive esophageal cancer.

Esophagectomy may be performed via open surgery or minimally invasive techniques, such as laparoscopic or robotic-assisted approaches, depending on the extent of disease, patient factors, and surgeon expertise.

2. **Surgical Approaches:**

Ivor Lewis Esophagectomy: A combination of abdominal and thoracic approaches, involving resection of the lower esophagus, stomach, and nearby lymph nodes, followed by reconstruction of the upper gastrointestinal tract with a gastric conduit.

Transhiatal Esophagectomy: An abdominal and cervical approach, involving resection of the lower esophagus and upper stomach through the abdomen, followed by creation of a cervical esophagogastric anastomosis.

3. **Postoperative Care and Outcomes:**

Esophagectomy is associated with significant perioperative risks and complications, including anastomotic leaks, pulmonary complications, and gastrointestinal dysfunction.

Postoperative care typically involves close monitoring in the intensive care unit (ICU), early initiation of enteral nutrition, and aggressive pulmonary hygiene to prevent complications.

Long-term outcomes of esophagectomy for esophagitis-related indications depend on various factors, including the extent of disease, tumor stage, surgical technique, and adjuvant therapy, with overall survival rates ranging from 50% to 70% at 5 years.

In summary, surgical management of esophagitis includes a range of procedures aimed at addressing underlying anatomical abnormalities, restoring the integrity of the gastroesophageal junction, and providing long-term relief from reflux symptoms. Fundoplication, endoscopic techniques, and esophagectomy are key surgical options for individuals with refractory symptoms, complications of reflux disease, or advanced esophageal pathology. The selection of surgical approach depends on individual patient factors, disease severity, and surgeon expertise, with the goal of optimizing outcomes and improving quality of life for individuals with esophagitis.

Preoperative Evaluation and Patient Selection

Preoperative evaluation and patient selection are critical steps in ensuring optimal outcomes and safety in individuals undergoing surgical management for esophagitis. A comprehensive assessment helps identify appropriate candidates for surgery, assesses the severity of esophageal disease, and determines the most suitable surgical approach based on individual patient factors and disease characteristics.

1. Comprehensive Clinical Evaluation:

- **Medical History:** Obtain a detailed medical history, including the duration and severity of symptoms, response to medical therapy, presence of complications (e.g., strictures, Barrett's esophagus), previous treatments, and comorbidities (e.g., obesity, diabetes, pulmonary disease).
- **Physical Examination:** Perform a thorough physical examination to assess for signs of esophageal disease, such as epigastric tenderness, abdominal distention, signs of malnutrition, or respiratory compromise.
- **Symptom Assessment:** Evaluate the nature and frequency of reflux symptoms (e.g., heartburn, regurgitation, dysphagia, chest pain), impact on quality of life, and response to medical therapy, including proton pump inhibitors (PPIs), histamine-2 receptor antagonists (H2RAs), and lifestyle modifications.

2. Diagnostic Testing:

- **Endoscopic Evaluation:** Perform esophagogastroduodenoscopy (EGD) with biopsies to assess the severity of esophagitis, presence of complications (e.g., strictures, Barrett's esophagus), and exclusion of other pathology (e.g., eosinophilic esophagitis, malignancy).
- **Esophageal Manometry:** Conduct esophageal manometry to evaluate esophageal motility, lower esophageal sphincter (LES) function, and assess for underlying motility disorders (e.g., achalasia, ineffective esophageal motility).

- **Ambulatory pH Monitoring:** Consider ambulatory pH monitoring to quantify acid reflux episodes, assess the frequency and duration of esophageal acid exposure, and determine the correlation between symptoms and reflux events.
- **Imaging Studies:** Order imaging studies such as barium swallow, computed tomography (CT) scan, or magnetic resonance imaging (MRI) to evaluate esophageal anatomy, identify hiatal hernias, assess for complications (e.g., strictures, perforation), and plan surgical approach.

3. Assessment of Surgical Candidacy:

- **Refractory Symptoms:** Individuals with persistent or recurrent symptoms of esophagitis despite optimal medical therapy, lifestyle modifications, and dietary interventions may be candidates for surgical intervention.
- **Complications of Reflux Disease:** Presence of complications such as esophageal strictures, Barrett's esophagus with dysplasia, or recurrent aspiration pneumonia may indicate the need for surgical correction to prevent disease progression and reduce the risk of long-term complications.
- **Response to Acid Suppression:** Evaluate the response to acid-suppressive medications (e.g., PPIs, H2RAs) and assess for adherence to medical therapy, frequency of breakthrough symptoms, and severity of esophageal inflammation to determine the appropriateness of surgical intervention.
- **Patient Preference and Goals:** Consider individual patient preferences, goals, and expectations regarding surgical treatment, including willingness to undergo surgery, acceptance of potential risks and

complications, and desire for long-term symptom relief and quality of life improvement.

4. Multidisciplinary Approach:

- **Collaborative Decision-Making:** Involve a multidisciplinary team of healthcare providers, including gastroenterologists, surgeons, dietitians, psychologists, and other specialists, in the preoperative evaluation and decision-making process.
- **Shared Decision-Making:** Engage patients in shared decision-making, providing information about treatment options, potential risks and benefits of surgery, and expected outcomes to facilitate informed decision-making and active participation in care.

5. Preoperative Optimization:

- **Medical Optimization:** Optimize medical management of esophagitis with acid-suppressive medications, lifestyle modifications (e.g., weight loss, dietary changes), and treatment of comorbid conditions (e.g., diabetes, hypertension) to improve perioperative outcomes and reduce postoperative complications.
- **Nutritional Assessment:** Conduct a nutritional assessment to identify and address malnutrition, micronutrient deficiencies, and nutritional risk factors, providing nutritional support and supplementation as needed to optimize perioperative nutrition and enhance recovery.

In summary, preoperative evaluation and patient selection are essential steps in identifying appropriate candidates for surgical management of esophagitis. A comprehensive assessment helps determine the severity of esophageal disease, evaluate treatment response, assess for complications, and involve patients in shared decision-making regarding surgical intervention. By conducting a thorough evaluation, involving multidisciplinary collaboration, and optimizing patients' medical and nutritional status, healthcare providers can ensure safe and successful surgical outcomes for individuals with esophagitis.

Printed in Great Britain
by Amazon